Managed Care
and Changing
Health Care Markets

Managed Care and Changing Health Care Markets

Michael A. Morrisey, editor

The AEI Press

Publisher for the American Enterprise Institute
WASHINGTON, D.C.

1998

Available in the United States from the AEI Press, c/o Publisher Resources Inc., 1224 Heil Quaker Blvd., P.O. Box 7001, La Vergne, TN 37086-7001; call toll free 1-800-269-6267. Distributed outside the United States by arrangement with Eurospan, 3 Henrietta Street, London WC2E 8LU England.

Library of Congress Cataloging-in-Publication Data

Managed care and changing health care markets / Michael Morrisey, editor.
    p. cm.
    Includes bibliographical references and index.
    ISBN 0-8447-4038-1 (cloth : alk. paper). — ISBN 0-8447-4039-X (paper : alk. paper)
    1. Managed care plans (Medical care)—United States.
2. Insurance, Health—United States. 3. Medical care—United States—Marketing. I. Morrisey, Michael A.
    RA412.2.M36 1998
    362.1'04258'0973—dc21   97-43998
                                                  CIP

1 3 5 7 9 10 8 6 4 2

THE AEI PRESS
Publisher for the American Enterprise Institute
1150 17th Street, N.W., Washington, D.C. 20036

Printed in the United States of America

Contents

8   THE EFFECTS OF HORIZONTAL HOSPITAL MERGERS ON
    NONMERGING HOSPITALS, *Robert A. Connor and Roger D.
    Feldman*   164

LIST OF TABLES

Foreword

In the past quarter-century, the American Enterprise Institute has published several major volumes that have provided in-depth analysis of a contemporary issue in health policy. In the 1970s, these volumes examined the use of certificate-of-need regulation of hospitals, the economics of medical malpractice, and national health insurance.[1] Several volumes in the 1980s covered the problem of rising health care costs and the effects of market competition.[2] Volumes in the early 1990s have concentrated on payment policies for physicians, health care reform, and the use of direct controls on health care expenditures.[3]

This volume, edited by Michael A. Morrisey, continues that tradition by looking at a set of issues that have dominated the health policy debate in the past few years, the unprecedented growth of managed care in health care markets. As Morrisey notes in his introduction, managed care has fundamentally changed the nature of health insurance and health delivery markets. All participants in health care markets, patients, providers, insurance companies, as well as health care institutions such as hospitals and health care plans, have been affected by these changes. The actual effects of these changes have been the subject of intense public debate, much of it political. While managed care has been credited with slowing the rise in health care expenditures, concerns have arisen about the effects of managed care on con-

---

1. See Clark C. Havighurst, *Regulating Health Facilities Construction* (Washington, D.C.: American Enterprise Institute, 1974); Simon Rottenberg, *The Economics of Medical Malpractice* (Washington, D.C.: American Enterprise Institute, 1978); and Mark V. Pauly, *National Health Insurance: What Now? What Later? What Never?* (Washington, D.C.: American Enterprise Institute, 1980).

2. See Mancur Olson, *A New Approach to the Economics of Health Care* (Washington, D.C.: American Enterprise Institute, 1981); and Jack A. Meyer, *Marke. Reforms in Health Care* (Washington, D.C.: American Enterprise Institute, 1983).

3. See H. E. Frech III, *Regulating Doctors' Fees: Competition, Benefits, and Controls under Medicare* (Washington, D.C.: AEI Press, 1991); Robert B. Helms, *American Health Policy: Critical Issues for Reform* (Washington, D.C.: AEI Press, 1993); and Robert B. Helms, *Health Policy Reform: Competition and Controls* (Washington, D.C.: AEI Press, 1993).

sumers' choices and the quality of care. Legislative proposals abound in state legislatures and in the U.S. Congress to increase substantially the government regulation of managed-care plans.

In the midst of the noisy political rhetoric issuing from the debate over managed care, this volume attempts to bring together a body of largely empirical research designed to add factual content and careful analysis to this continuing debate. Professor Morrisey has assembled a set of the country's leading health economists and edited their research into a comprehensive but readable volume. AEI wishes to thank Professor Morrisey and the authors of these chapters for their hard work and the high professional standards exhibited in this research. The public debate about managed care is far from over, but perhaps research of this type will help to focus that debate on the important issues.

ROBERT B. HELMS
Director, Health Policy Studies
American Enterprise Institute

Acknowledgments

Thanks are due, first, to Bob Helms for proposing this venture and assisting in every step of its development. He is a wonderful organizer and facilitator and a gentle critic. Thanks are also due to the American Enterprise Institute and its staff for the rapid and careful production of the book. I am also grateful to a diligent reviewer who carefully critiqued all the chapters, which were revised in response to his comments. The product is much better for this review. Thanks, of course, are also due to the authors—a stronger collection of scholars would be hard to find. Each enthusiastically agreed to participate, many changing already full schedules to accommodate this book. The chapters are not only relevant, rigorous, and well written, but they were uniformly delivered on time. There is nothing more an editor can hope for than quality and timeliness.

Finally, thanks are due to the foundations and agencies that sponsored the research on which these studies are based. The Agency for Health Care Policy and Research funded the Connor-Feldman work on hospital mergers and the Simon-White-Born-Dranove analysis of physician markets. The Robert Wood Johnson Foundation funded the analysis underlying the Gaynor and Haas-Wilson work on vertical integration and the Dowd-Feldman examination of level dollar contributions to employee health plans. The Henry J. Kaiser Family Foundation funded the work underlying the Jensen-Morrisey analysis of small group insurance markets. Analyses of this sort are public goods in the classic economic sense of that term. These organizations improve the policy process by investing in understanding of how health care markets function.

Contributors

MICHAEL A. MORRISEY is professor of health economics in the School of Public Health at the University of Alabama at Birmingham and director of the UAB Lister Hill Center for Health Policy. The author of two books and over ninety articles on health economics and health policy issues, his research focuses on managed care. In addition to work on the small-group insurance market, Mr. Morrisey's current research includes a project on managed care and hospital-physician integration, funded by the Agency for Health Care Policy Research, and an examination of hospital contracting with managed care and the effects of any-willing-provider laws, funded by the Robert Wood Johnson Foundation.

PATRICIA BORN is an assistant professor in the Department of Finance, Insurance, Real Estate, and Health Systems at the University of Connecticut. She was previously employed in the Center for Health Policy Research at the American Medical Association and taught at DePaul University in Chicago, Illinois. Her current research activities include the evaluation of the influence of managed care on the distribution of physician earnings and analysis of the financial performance of health maintenance organizations.

ROBERT A. CONNOR is an associate professor in the Department of Health Care Management at the University of Minnesota. He was associate director for patient services at Strong Memorial Hospital of the University of Rochester. Mr. Connor's research focuses on geographic access to health care, health care mergers and antitrust policy, financing and management of population-based health care delivery systems, and insurance purchasing decisions and market dynamics. He has contributed to *Academic Medicine, Computers in Healthcare, DRG Monitor, Health Care Management Review, Hospital & Health Services Administration, Journal of Economic Psychology, Journal of Public Budgeting and Financial Management, Journal of Health Economics, Journal of Long Term Care Administration, Medical Care, Medical Care Review,* and *Topics in Health Care Financing.*

BRYAN DOWD is a professor in the Division of Health Services Research and Policy in the School of Public Health at the University of Minnesota and director of graduate studies for the master's of science program in health services research and policy. He teaches advanced health services research methods in the doctoral and master's programs offered through the institute. Mr. Dowd is a member of the health services research study section of the Agency for Health Care Policy and Research. He is an author, with Roger Feldman and Jon Christianson, of *Competitive Pricing for Medicare* (AEI Press, 1996).

DAVID DRANOVE is the Richard Paget Distinguished Professor of Management and Strategy and chair of the Department of Management and Strategy at Northwestern University's Kellogg School of Management. He is also professor of health services management. Before joining Kellogg, Mr. Dranove was on the faculty of the University of Chicago Graduate School of Business. Mr. Dranove is a founding partner of the Health Economics Practice Group and an affiliate of the Law and Economics Consulting Group. Mr. Dranove has contributed to six books, is coauthor of the textbook *The Economics of Strategy*, and is lead author on over fifty research papers and monographs. He is the author, with William White, of *Clinton's Specialist Quota: Shaky Premises, Questionable Consequences* (AEI Press, 1994).

ROGER D. FELDMAN is the Blue Cross Professor of Health Insurance at the University of Minnesota. He directed one of the four national research centers sponsored by the Health Care Financing Administration and was a senior staff member of the Council of Economic Advisers, where he was lead author of one chapter of the *1985 Economic Report of the President*. Mr. Feldman is on the editorial board of *Inquiry* and is a regular contributor to health services research and economics journals. Mr. Feldman is the author, with Bryan Dowd and Jon Christianson, of *Competitive Pricing for Medicare* (AEI Press, 1996). He is currently working on a study of horizontal mergers among hospitals.

MARTIN GAYNOR holds the E. J. Barone Chair in Health Systems Management and is an associate professor of economics and public policy in the H. John Heinz III School of Public Policy and Management and the Graduate School of Industrial Administration at Carnegie Mellon University. He is also a research associate of the National Bureau of Economic Research in Cambridge, Massachusetts. Mr. Gaynor taught at Johns Hopkins University and a number of other universities and was a visitor at the Hungarian Academy of Sciences in 1991. He is a member of the health services research study section of the Agency for Health Care Policy Research and is on the editorial board of *Health Services Research*. He has contributed to *Journal of Political Economy*, *RAND Journal of Economics*, *Journal of Human Resources*, *Economics Letters*, *Journal of Economics and Management Strategy*, *Public Choice*, and other publications.

DEBORAH HAAS-WILSON is an associate professor of economics at Smith College. She was a member of the health services research study section of the Agency for Health Care Policy and Research. Ms. Haas-Wilson was a member of the executive committee of the health economics committee of the American Public Health Association. She has testified before state legislative committees and served as a witness in numerous court cases. Ms. Haas-Wilson's research focuses on the economics of regulation in markets characterized by informational asymmetries.

GAIL A. JENSEN is an associate professor at Wayne State University, jointly appointed in the university's Institute of Gerontology and Department of Economics. Much of her research over the past ten years has focused on issues surrounding markets for private health insurance in the United States, particularly employer-sponsored group coverage. Ms. Jensen has published studies on the content and changing nature of employer-sponsored health benefits, including the growth of managed care, the scope of corporate health benefits for retirees, the changing views of employers regarding health care reform, and the effects of state insurance regulations on employer insurance offerings.

ADAM MEIROWITZ received a Master of Science degree in public policy analysis from the University of Rochester. He is working on a Ph.D. in economics at Stanford.

CAROL J. SIMON is an associate professor at the School of Public Health and the Institute of Government and Public Affairs at the University of Illinois at Chicago. She has taught at the University of California at Los Angeles and the University of Chicago. Ms. Simon's current areas of research include the impact of managed care on physicians, the introduction and effect of any-willing-provider laws on physicians, and physician involvement in Medicaid.

WILLIAM D. WHITE is a professor in the Department of Economics and the Institute of Government and Public Affairs at the University of Illinois at Chicago. His major areas of research include the impact of managed care on hospital and physician markets, payment system design, and professional regulation.

JACK ZWANZIGER is an associate professor in the Department of Community and Preventive Medicine at the University of Rochester. He is also the director of the doctoral program in health services research. Mr. Zwanziger was a lecturer at the University of California at Los Angeles, a manager of the Telecommunications Policy Office of the Ontario Ministry of Transportation and Communications, and a senior policy analyst in the Policy Analysis and Coordination Office in the same department. His research interests include the effect of managed care and competition on provider behavior.

1
Introduction

Michael A. Morrisey

The past decade has seen the remarkable growth of managed care. As recently as 1985 only 7.5 percent of insured workers had coverage through an HMO (Jensen et al. 1987). The term *preferred provider organization* (PPO) was just entering the vocabulary of health care professionals; a tally of the number of people eligible for such plans was not yet being considered. Employees of small firms almost never had coverage through a managed-care plan. By 1995 managed care had become the insurance mechanism of choice for private sector workers; 73 percent of workers in firms of *all* sizes were covered through a managed-care plan (Jensen et al. 1997). The term *PPO* is now a common one, although *point of service plan* gives pause to the uninitiated. Virtually all the states are experimenting with managed care in their Medicaid programs. Medicare reformers rely heavily on the concept.

Managed care has not merely changed the name on the insurance card of many Americans. It is beginning to change fundamentally the nature of health insurance and health care delivery markets. Once we routinely worried about runaway health care costs. Double-digit increases in insurance premiums were common. As figure 1–1 shows, however, the rates of increase in health insurance premiums have declined steadily since 1989. In 1995 and 1996 they were below the rate of general inflation as measured by the consumer price index. Private sector health insurance premiums actually declined in real terms! Pundits have argued that recent declines in the profitability of many managed-care firms will lead to a new round of escalating premiums. Well-respected students of the market, however, have publicly disagreed, arguing instead that efforts to raise premiums significantly will be met with shifts by employers to other managed-care firms (CSHSC 1997). Ten years ago, even five years ago, no credible academic or market participant would have made such a claim.

The move to managed care has spawned all sorts of changes. The once dominant indemnity insurance plans now have only a quarter of the private health insurance market. Small employers are now almost

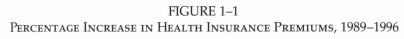

FIGURE 1–1
Percentage Increase in Health Insurance Premiums, 1989–1996

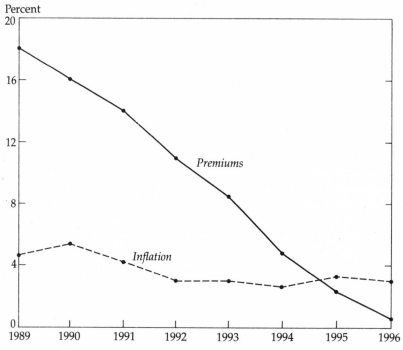

Source: Jensen et al. (1997) and CSHSC (1997).

as likely as large ones to offer a managed-care plan. Employers are finding ways to structure premium sharing to allow workers to see the savings from choosing less expensive plans. Hospitals are competing on a price basis. Providers who once complained about how poorly Medicaid pays now worry about losing their Medicaid contract. Specialists have seen their incomes decline—despite all their supposed ability to induce demand. Where once we worried that hospitals would not work cooperatively, now we worry that consolidation in the industry will give networks of providers too much market power. We are even beginning to rethink what we mean by a health care market.

The purpose of this book is to explore the effects of managed care—of selective contracting—on insurance and health care markets. While the growth of managed care has been dramatic, the growth in the rhetoric surrounding these changes has been even more dramatic. Here we present new research, predominantly empirical, examining several of the key issues surrounding managed care. Some of the findings are surprising, such as the extent of premium expenditures that are saved when employers set a level dollar limit on their pretax contribution to health insurance. Others are less surprising, such as the extent to which managed care has reduced physician income. Still others are controversial, such as the view that one should look at competition among networks rather than among their constituent parts. Through each of the studies the intent is to reduce the rhetoric by rigorously examining the issues, either empirically or conceptually. Each of the chapters has been subject to external blinded peer review. Unlike the academic journals, however, these chapters are intended to be accessible to a policy audience.

The book is organized into three parts. The first deals with managed care and employers, the second with providers, and the third examines issues of market definition and horizontal and vertical integration—the formation of provider networks and the linking of insurance and health care delivery services. In the remainder of this introduction, I will set the stage by summarizing the studies and putting them in the context of the existing research.

Managed Care

Arguably the engine of all this change has been "managed care." The term has taken on a variety of meanings. To some it means capitation; providers are paid a fixed amount per subscriber for all or some well-defined component of their care. But capitation is relatively rare in the hospital setting Morrisey et al. (1996) and Hillman et al. (1992) have clearly demonstrated that even capitated HMOs do not necessarily pay their physicians on a capitated basis. Others have argued that managed care means any plan that manages the utilization of its members. Under this definition indemnity plans that included pre-hospital admission certification would be managed-care plans. It is not obvious that managed-care plans are necessarily a subset of insurance firms, since many PPOs do not bear any underwriting risk; they simply administer a set of contracts between employer-purchasers and provider-sellers.

From my perspective, the most useful definition of managed care is an arrangement by which buyers selectively contract for services with providers. The key is that some providers get contracts and some do not. As long as price can be a factor in the negotiations, the sorts of changes we see in insurance and health care markets are reasonably predictable. Competition to be among the selected tends to drive prices to marginal costs, tends to make providers look for consolidations that reduce costs, and tends to lead providers to find ways to acquire and maintain market power. It also leads managed-care firms to find that level of amenities, clinical quality, and mix of providers that attracts subscribers.

In some sense the potential of selective contracting was always understood. Justin Kimbel is usually credited with founding the first hospital insurance plan. At the beginning of the depression, accounts receivable were way up at his Baylor Hospital in Texas. He hit upon charging employees of the Dallas school district fifty cents per month for hospital care *at his hospital* should they become ill. Within a half-dozen years the American Hospital Association and its Hospital Service Plan Commission, the forerunner of Blue Cross, was approving hospital insurance plans. Initially single-hospital plans like Kimbel's were approved, as were communitywide, "freedom-of-choice" plans that allowed for care at any hospital in a community. By 1936 only communitywide plans were being approved. As Rufus Rorem, the chair of the Hospital Service Plan Commission, is reported to have commented, the early single-hospital plans had resulted in "competition among the hospitals, and interference with the subscribers' freedom of choice, and the physicians' prerogatives in the care of private patients" (Starr 1982). Given the research, it would appear that Rorem had it right about competition.

Managed Care and Employers

Much of the research on employer-sponsored health insurance, at least as it relates to managed care, has focused on two themes: first, the sensitivity of workers to changes in out-of-pocket premiums, and second, biased selection among workers when faced with multiple-plan options. It is also the case that virtually all the research has focused on larger firms.

Biased selection and worker price sensitivity are key to understanding the development of managed care over the past decade. One can think of a large firm as having workers with a range of preferences for and against the limited panel of providers and the style of practice that is common in a managed-care firm. Other things equal, when an employer offers both a managed-care plan and an indemnity plan, some will prefer the managed-care plan and the remainder will select the indemnity. There is an impressive body of literature that suggests that those choosing the managed-care plan tend to be low utilizers in whatever plan they enroll in. See Miller and Luft (1994) for a recent review. Consistent with this research, the recent ProPAC (1996) analysis of Medicare risk (HMO) contracts concluded that the method Medicare uses to pay HMOs overpays, because it fails to account for self-selected Medicare-HMO beneficiaries' tendency to use fewer services regardless of plan.

Many have argued that the recent profitability of managed-care plans stemmed from their ability to attract lower utilizers and to charge employers prices akin to those charged by the indemnity plans, so-called shadow pricing. Under this scenario the combined health insurance bill presented to the employer is higher, not lower, and the managed-care plan is indeed very profitable.

This profitability, however, will only be transitory in the face of selective contracting *and* price sensitivity on the part of workers and their employers. Selective contracting allows other organizations to put together their own insurance or delivery plans to be offered to workers along with the existing indemnity and managed-care product or in place of the existing managed-care plan. Then, if workers are sensitive to premium differences, they will switch from one managed-care firm to another, and potentially from the indemnity plan to a managed-care product. Indeed, one should expect an employer to drop one managed-care product and add another if workers sufficiently value the lower premiums.[1]

So, how price sensitive are workers? Early empirical work by Welch (1986) investigated the extent to which workers were willing to switch from an indemnity plan to an HMO as the relative premiums changed. He found that a 10 percent increase in the monthly out-of-pocket premium had a short-run effect of reducing the HMO share of enrolled workers by 2 percent. The long-run effect was a 5 percent reduction. Long et al. (1988) demonstrated that the number of options available to workers mattered. Controlling for other factors, a $5 increase in an HMO's relative premium increased disenrollment by 66.7 percent. A $5 increase in the relative premium resulted in approximately 70 disenrollments per 1,000 subscribers when there were five HMOs offered by the firm, but only 58 disenrollments per 1,000 when there were three plans.

---

1. One might object that the key issue is the employer's price sensitivity. As a matter of theory, the employer's price responsiveness is much less important. Health insurance is provided in the workplace because workers value it and are willing to trade monetary wages for it. In a sense, health insurance in the employment setting is a derived demand on the part of employers for a means of employee compensation. As with all derived demands, the greater the elasticity of demand for the product, the greater the elasticity of demand for the input. Thus, the greater the price sensitivity of workers for health insurance, the greater the employer's price sensitivity for employer-sponsored coverage. As an empirical matter, there have been few studies that have directly addressed the extent of employer price sensitivity for health insurance.

More recent work by Feldman et al. (1989) and Dowd and Feldman (1994) carefully considered the precise nature of the options workers actually had available to them. They found that workers were enormously willing to move from one similar-style plan to another, from one HMO to another, for example, and less price responsive when moving from one plan type to another. For workers with single coverage in a firm and several plan options, a 1 percent increase in the out-of-pocket premium of an HMO was associated with a 7.9 percent reduction in the probability of selecting that plan.

Buchmueller and Feldstein (1996) report on a natural experiment that shows the dramatic propensity of workers to change plans for very modest increases in out-of-pocket premiums. In 1993 the faculty and staff of the University of California system paid no out-of-pocket premium for any of the managed-care plans, or for any but the high-option indemnity plan offered through the UC system. In 1994 the UC system switched to a model of level-dollar contributions in which faculty and staff would pay no out-of-pocket premium for the lowest-cost plan, but would pay the full extra premium for any plan they selected that had a higher premium. The results of this policy change are shown in figure 1–2. When faced with a $10 per month increase in out-of-pocket premiums, more than 25 percent of faculty and staff switched plans. When faced with greater out-of-pocket premium increases, even larger proportions of workers switched.

This enormous price sensitivity is the driving force behind the changes that we have observed in health care over the past decade. Given the opportunity to purchase on basis of price, purchasers do so. Insurers are driven to set premiums at marginal cost and to look for ways to cut their costs. Pretty quickly hospitals, physicians, and other health care providers are forced to do the same.

This sets the stage for chapter 2 of this volume. There Bryan Dowd and Roger Feldman investigate the use of the level-dollar contribution by employers. Advocates like Alain Enthoven have long argued that employers should do what the University of California system did in 1994. That is, they should offer several plans and require workers to pay the full marginal cost of any plan they select over and above the least costly plan. This allows workers to reap the savings of any lower-cost plan they select.

Dowd and Feldman essentially raise two questions. First, how much money, if any, is saved by adopting a strategy of level-dollar minimum-premium contributions? Second, given the conceptual superiority of this strategy and the empirical evidence of its cost savings, why do more firms not use it? They answer the first question and offer some evidence and important speculation on the second.

FIGURE 1–2

PERCENTAGE OF ALL EMPLOYEES AND HMO ENROLLEES SWITCHING
HEALTH PLANS BY INCREASE IN MONTHLY CONTRIBUTIONS,
1993–1994

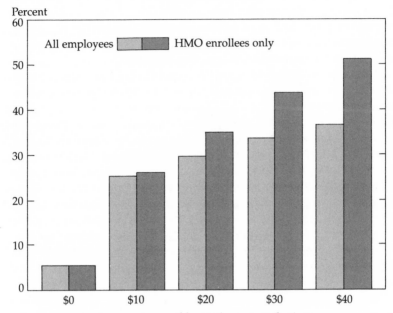

Increase in monthly employee contributions

SOURCE: Buchmueller and Feldstein (1996).

Based on recent employer surveys, level-dollar contributions to
employee health benefit plans are relatively rare; only about 14 percent
of firms are reported to use this approach. Governmental units are
much more likely to do so. Consequently, Dowd and Feldman surveyed 318 large city and county governments in 1994, collecting data
on a series of health insurance issues. Approximately 35 percent of big
cities and counties use some variant of the level-dollar approach. Only
about half of these, however, set the level-dollar amount at the level of
the least costly plan for single coverage. Only a quarter do so for family
coverage. Moreover, more than 30 percent pay the full premium for all
plan options.

The answer to the first question is clear from their study. After
using a variety of econometric techniques to control for other factors
and to account for the firm's decision to use level-dollar methods in
the first place, Dowd and Feldman conclude that "the failure to pay
a level-dollar contribution is estimated to increase single and family

7

coverage premiums by roughly 7–8 percent." When employers use a level-dollar approach, insurers are faced with the full price sensitivity of workers, and as a consequence average premiums are lower. This provides some important guidance to workers and their employers. Their health care costs can be reduced significantly when level-dollar contributions are used.

The second question is in some ways more interesting. If premiums can be reduced by 7–8 percent, why have more employers not adopted this approach? A simple answer is that neither employers nor their workers knew that such savings could be had. Perhaps this is true, but ordinarily economists argue that when large numbers of firms consistently do something over time, there is usually a good reason for that behavior. Dowd and Feldman argue that one important reason that firms may not use level-dollar contributions is the concern that there are significant differences in the health status across enrollees of the plans offered. Indeed, one of the few variables that predict the use of level-dollar methods in their study is one that indicates that the employer thought there was an unequal distribution of risk across plans. This leads to a further question: Why would the employer care? One answer is, concern over fairness for his workers. But this is seldom a comfortable answer for economists. Another answer, more consistent with economic theory, is that those people who choose the more generous plans are somehow more productive workers. If so, the apparent subsidy to these workers would be economically justified. There is some evidence that married workers are more productive than singles, for example, and one can build a case that over the life cycle of employment with a firm, younger workers are willing to be systematically underpaid knowing they will be somewhat overpaid in later years. Like pensions, this sort of compensation structure binds the worker to the firm. Given the results of this chapter, we need to know more about why firms do not use level-dollar contributions. If we do not understand the issues better, we set up the unintended consequences that policy watchers always eschew.

Chapter 3 in this volume is also concerned with managed care in the employer setting. The bulk of research on employer-sponsored health insurance has focused on large employers. But much of the concern about the uninsured has focused on small employers. There is a strong perception that small employers are increasingly not sponsoring coverage and that managed care has not made significant inroads into the small-group market. Moreover, the states have enacted a number of laws dealing with issues of insurance underwriting, bare-bones provisions, and pricing limitations designed to make insurance more available to small-group purchasers, if not necessarily less expensive.

Gail Jensen and Michael Morrisey examine these issues, reporting new results on the nature of the insurance coverage offered through small employers and summarizing the results of two of their just-completed studies on the small-group market. Two themes stand out.

First, the move to managed care by employers with fewer than fifty workers has been as dramatic as it has been rapid. Among small firms providing health insurance, the proportion of workers covered by a managed-care plan increased from 27 percent in 1993 to 70 percent in 1995. In many ways this is a much more significant change than that observed in large employers, because virtually all small firms offer only a single benefit plan. Offering a managed-care product in a small-firm context means giving up indemnity coverage.

The authors argue that large employers have played a key role in this conversion. Everyone knows someone in the office who might be called "the shopper." He or she searches out the best value on VCRs and computers; the rest of us observe and try to do the same. It appears that large employers have implicitly played this role for small employers. In continuing to offer managed-care products they have essentially "certified" the concept of managed care, if not the particular firms. With a lag, small employers follow suit. This finding has important policy implications. It suggests that managed care is not limited to markets with lots of large firms. Rather, while large firms lead, small firms follow. Those markets that have not yet seen significant managed-care penetration, because of a limited number of large employers, nonetheless, can expect to see development in their communities, as the experience of the few larger employers spreads to the smaller firms.

Jensen and Morrisey also demonstrate that price matters in the switch to managed care. Relative to conventional coverage, a 10 percent lower premium in 1995 was associated with a 3.3 percent increase in the probability that a small firm would offer a managed-care product. This price responsiveness is much lower than that reported in studies of workers—but those studies examined changes from one managed-care plan to another. Here the switch is from an indemnity plan to managed care. Even the worker-level studies suggest that there is much less price sensitivity when switching across plan type. It is also important to note that this price sensitivity may reflect the sort of paradigm shift that advocates have expected. In their 1993 data the authors found no statistically significant effect of price. By 1995 it is strong, although relatively small. Efforts of insurers to raise prices may be hard to sustain in the new environment.

The second theme of the Jensen and Morrisey chapter is the growth in the provision of health insurance coverage through small employers. In 1991, only 34 percent of small employers sponsored health insurance for their employees. By 1995, however, 53 percent sponsored coverage. Using small-employer data from the 1989–1995 period, they demonstrate that coverage is cyclical, rising and falling with the general economy. One means of increasing the propensity of small firms to offer coverage is to maintain a strong, growing economy. In many ways it *is* "the economy, stupid."

During this period, some forty-five states enacted laws dealing with limitations on preexisting conditions, and thirty-eight states enacted laws requiring insurers to issue coverage to any firm willing to pay the premium. Additional laws dealt with so-called bare-bones laws that exempted small employers from state mandated–benefits laws. In general, these laws did little to expand coverage among workers in small firms. Guaranteed issue laws, however, which require an insurer to cover any firm willing to pay the premiums, did increase the propensity of the smallest of small firms to sponsor coverage. Their propensity to do so increased by eight percentage points.

Jensen and Morrisey suggest that the key to the provision of health insurance by small employers is price. If workers and the employers are to buy coverage, prices must fall. This is clear from attitudinal surveys of small employers and from the empirical studies of price sensitivity among workers. Figure 1–1 suggested that insurance premiums had been increasing less rapidly over the past several years. If market forces can lead to actually *lower* premiums, there is hope for further increases in the number of small employers sponsoring coverage.

Managed Care and Providers

One might view the late 1970s and early 1980s as the golden age of American hospitals, at least from the hospitals' perspective. Cost-based reimbursement was paramount; patients and payers seemed unconcerned about the price of care. Robinson and Luft (1985) explored the nature of hospital competition over this period. Controlling for other factors, they found that hospitals in communities with more hospitals had higher costs. This is exactly the opposite conclusion one would expect from simple economic theory. The explanation is straightforward. Since price was not a significant issue, hospitals competed for physicians and patients along dimensions that did matter: services, amenities, and quality. More competitors meant that competition along these dimensions was more intense and costs were higher.

This circumstance existed in California as well. In 1983, however, the state legislature enacted two laws that introduced selective contracting. First, it gave its Medicaid agency the ability to negotiate with hospitals and to enter into contracts only with a limited number of them. Second, it made clear that payers could contract only with selected hospitals if they chose, and could deny contracts to others.

Zwanziger and Melnick (1988) examined the rates of change in hospital costs before and after the enactment of these laws. In the 1980–1982 period, before enactment, hospitals with more competitors had annual cost increases of 6.6 percent; those with fewer competitors had increases of 5.5 percent. After the enactment of the laws, during the 1983–1985 period, those hospitals with more competitors had cost *reductions* of nearly 1 percent, but the hospitals in less competitive areas had increases of 2.8 percent. The suggestion is clearly that selective contracting made price as well as services, amenities, and quality part of the negotiation.

In subsequent work Melnick et al. (1992) were given access to a measure of the actual transaction prices negotiated by a large California PPO with hospitals throughout the state. They found that the transaction prices reflected standard economic factors. When there were more hospitals in the market, the PPO was able to negotiate lower prices. When the PPO had a larger share of the hospital's book of business, the PPO got a still lower price. When the hospital had only a small share of the PPO's subscribers, the hospital got a lower price. Moreover, even controlling for these factors, the PPO was able to negotiate a still lower price if a given hospital or any of the hospitals in its market area had low occupancy. Taken together these studies provide the strongest evidence to date that selective contracting changes the nature of provider markets. Price matters, and conventional market forces work to drive prices down.

This raises the question of which providers get the contracts. Heretofore there has been but one study of that issue. Feldman et al. (1990) examined contractual arrangements made by six HMOs in four unnamed (non-California) markets. As table 1–1 shows, the HMOs did not contract with all local hospitals. In fact, only 10 to 47 percent of hospitals got contracts.

The team tried to explain which hospitals were selected based on such factors as price, quality, and location. Methodologically, this is not an easy exercise. Location is relatively easy to measure, quality is enormously difficult. Price is problematic. Ideally one would like to know what prices were actually offered by all the hospitals in the community. But it is virtually impossible to get prices that never resulted in contracts. The study team used hospital costs as a measure of price and used characteristics of the hospital such as having a teaching program, ownership, and the number of services offered as proxy measures for quality. What they found was that price *was not* a statistically

11

TABLE 1–1
HOSPITAL USE IN AN HMO MARKET AREA

City	HMO	HMO Type	Hospitals in Area	Hospitals Used	Percentage of Hospitals Used
1	A	Staff	71	7	10
	B	IPA	107	46	43
2	C	Staff	36	8	22
3	D	Network	32	15	47
	E	Network	33	8	25
4	F	IPA	53	18	34

SOURCE: Feldman et al. (1990).

significant determinant of which hospitals got contracts. Instead, their proxy quality measures were the only statistically meaningful determinants. Those hospitals that had teaching programs and were not public general hospitals were more likely to get the contracts.

Feldman and his colleagues went further, to examine which hospitals get the patient volume, given a contract. In this analysis they deal only with contract hospitals, and so have available the actual prices negotiated. What they find in this portion of the study is that price matters tremendously. For staff and network HMOs, a $1 higher price at a hospital is associated with a 3 percent lower volume. Even the independent practice association–style HMOs (IPAs) appear to be able to "channel" patients. For them a hospital with a $1 higher price gets a 1 percent lower volume. This study suggests that "quality" gets the contract for a hospital, but price gets the volume.

Chapter 4 by Jack Zwanziger and Adam Meirowitz is only the second study to examine the issue of which hospitals get managed-care contracts. They use 1993 survey data from thirteen metropolitan areas to revisit the first half of the Feldman et al. study. Unlike the earlier work, however, they have information on PPOs as well as HMOs. The findings reinforce much of the earlier work, but also offer some important new insights.

First, managed-care firms contracted with a limited set of providers—on average across the markets, with about 45 percent of hospitals. The range was from a single hospital to 88 percent of all the hospitals in the market. HMOs tended to have smaller networks than PPOs, and older plans tended to have smaller networks. This is consistent with the major tenet of selective contracting—only some providers get contracts. There is also a suggestion that as managed-care plans mature, they prune their networks. Obviously, multiyear studies are needed to confirm this directly.

Second, price, or more precisely costs per admission, exhibited an inverted U-shaped relationship with the probability of having a contract. The hospitals in the lowest quartile of costs were about 30 percent less likely to get contracts. Those hospitals with the highest costs were 20 percent less likely to get contracts than were the hospitals in the middle of the cost distribution. From the results, it would appear that managed-care plans have as much difficulty in measuring quality as do researchers. They appear to be avoiding high-cost hospitals, presumably out of concern over costs, but also avoiding the lowest cost hospitals, perhaps out of a concern for inferior quality. Future research carefully measuring clinical quality and consumer perceptions of quality is needed.

Third, the characteristics of hospitals with and without contracts offer a fascinating insight into market behavior. Zwanziger and Meirowitz found that public general hospitals were less likely to get contracts than were nonprofit institutions. This is no surprise, given the perception that quality of care may be lower there. But for-profit hospitals are even less likely than public generals to have contracts. This may be a reflection of perceived quality, but it flies in the face of well-publicized conversions of nonprofit to for-profit hospitals. Moreover, Zwanziger and Meirowitz found no evidence that hospitals that were part of systems were any more likely to get managed-care contracts. This may be an artifact of the broad definition of system membership that the authors were compelled to use. Some systems are local, composed of hospitals in a single market or a relatively small region. Others are national or regional in scope. If the relevant market is a single metropolitan area, a local system may have an advantage in offering services to a managed-care firm—as suggested by chapter 6 in this volume. A national system may not have such an advantage. Combining both sorts of systems may lead to a finding of no effect. In either event, the results should give some pause to those seeking to expand hospital systems as a managed-care strategy. In general, however, those examining hospital contracting behavior must pay greater attention to measures of quality and to the dynamic nature of the contractual relationships.

There has been almost no empirical work examining nonhospital providers. One might extrapolate, however, that the effects of selective contracting found in hospital markets would also apply to physician and other medical markets. If so, one would expect that managed-care firms have contracted with only a subset of the available physicians in any given market. One would expect that selective contracting had reduced physician prices. One would also suspect that because physicians are more mobile than hospitals, they may have moved away from areas where managed care is more prevalent. There is good evidence that physicians' choice of specialty is very responsive to expected lifetime earnings. Those specialties that offer higher returns on educational investment attract more residents. Thus, if managed care has changed the demand for various specialists, one would expect that lifetime earnings would be changed and there would be a movement on the part of new residents away from "declining" specialties and into "growing" ones.

In chapter 5 of this volume, Carol Simon and her colleagues William White, Patricia Born, and David Dranove continue their examinations of physician markets under managed care. In addition to summarizing and expanding their findings with respect to physician incomes, they also explore the effects that managed care has had on locational choice and residency specialty choice.

As with all studies of physicians, distinctions must be made among specialties. Simon and company examine primary care physicians, hospital-based physicians, and medical and surgical specialists. They use data from the 1985 to 1994 period, focusing particularly on the changes that took place in 1994.

Taken together, the results suggest substantial market level effects on the relative incomes of physicians. First, controlling for other factors, the incomes of primary care physicians grew most rapidly over much of the period in markets with high managed-care penetration. This is consistent with the increased reliance on primary care in managed-care firms. Second, the incomes of hospital-based physicians grew least rapidly in markets with high managed-care penetration. This may be a reflection of managed care's effect on hospitals as much as it is on physician markets directly. Third, the incomes of medical and surgical subspecialists also lagged in the markets with the highest managed-care penetration, although these results were not as statistically significant. Moreover, in the 1993–1994 period, with one exception, the incomes of all physician groups fell the most in markets with the highest degree of managed-care penetration. The story appears very similar to that of hospital markets, where selective contracting slowed the rate of increase in costs. These physician numbers, however, undoubtedly understate the effects of managed care. The Simon results are marketwide. Selective contracting would suggest that it is those physicians without contracts who would have seen the greatest declines in their incomes.

For the most part, the locational decisions were consistent with the income results. Hospital-based physicians appeared most responsive to the incentives. States with the highest managed-care growth had the smallest increases in physician-to-population ratios over the period. A similar pattern held for subspecialists, although not nearly so dramatically. Surprisingly, primary care ratios have not been rising as rapidly in highly penetrated managed-care markets as would be suggested by the income numbers. The authors suggest that this lower rate of increase may be caused by managed-care firms' tending to locate and grow in areas where there are greater numbers of competing providers. But if this is so, one would not have expected to see the income increases. It is conceivable that the substitution of nonphysicians and the shift of specialists into more nonspecialty care may be absorbing the increased demand. Clearly, however, more work in this area is needed.

Finally, Simon et al. report on the residency matching program over the 1989 to 1997 period. Here they find that family practice residency programs expanded from a low of 1,636 slots in 1993 to 3,262 in 1997. Moreover, the fill-rate increased from 59.8 percent in 1989 to more than 71 percent in 1997. Positions and fill-rates for pediatricians expanded over the period as well. Consistent with the incentives implied by the changes in real income, the number of hospital-based physician positions and their fill-rates have declined since 1993. Surgical specialty positions and fill-rates both increased in 1997 after declining in the preceding years. The residency decisions are consistent with the relative increase in primary care income and decline in hospital-based incomes. The surgical results are not inconsistent with the more muddled story on specialist income. In general, the results suggest that managed care is affecting physician income and leading to changes in the location and specialty choices of physicians.

Antitrust and Managed Care

The purpose of the antitrust laws is to promote competition. The general theory is a straightforward structure-and-performance argument. More competition tends to enhance consumer well-being by pushing prices down to marginal cost. Given similar products and cost structures, having more competitors implies having more competition. The issues arise in the application of this simple theory. How many competitors are enough? Are costs really the same, or are there significant economies of scale in production that would outweigh the concerns about competition? More esoteric issues revolve around the definitions of the product and the market. Are aluminum foil and plastic wrap essentially the same product as viewed by consumers? If they are, the merger of the largest aluminum foil suppliers may have no effect on the food wrap market. If they are not, the merger may decrease competition and raise prices. Are Seattle and Tacoma in the same market? If so, a merger of milk distributors in Tacoma may not lessen competition; if they are not, it may.

Each industry tends to have its own special features that further complicate the application of the antitrust principles. In banking, is the product residential loans or does it include commercial loans as well? Are credit cards part of the same product? Is the market one of residential loans in Nashville, or is it the price of credit in Tennessee? Do automated teller machines allow fewer competitors to exert competition over a larger geographic area?

Health care has its own set of complexities, not the least of which is a history of cost-based reimbursement and, as Dranove, Shanley, and White (1993) have argued, competition that was driven by the patient rather than the payer. I noted above that a lack of concern over price led to competition along the dimensions of services, quality, and amenities. This implies some difficulties in applying the structure-and-performance model. More competitors led to higher costs and higher prices. So, does a merger of two hospitals result in enhanced competition or reduced consumer welfare?

The move to selective contracting and payer-driven competition in health care makes the structure-and-performance model more easily applicable to health care. Now a key decision maker has the incentive to view both the services-quality-amenities and the price. As we have seen, the empirical evidence increasingly tends to support a view that more competitors, at least in hospital markets, is associated with lower prices for managed-care firms. New challenges, however, also emerge with the growth of managed care. First, the nature of the relevant product is changing. Patients are no longer buying insurance or physician, hospital, pharmacy, and dentist services in distinct product markets. Increasingly they are buying a package that contains all these products. On the one hand, this implies that the antitrust concern will focus on whether there is competition among the suppliers of the packages. On the other hand, the nature of the buyers of services in the insurance, physician, hospital, pharmacy, and dental markets is changing. Does this enhance competition, or does it give new market power to providers? Moreover, the "packages" often come about by combinations of formerly distinct providers—networks of hospitals, for example. Does this sort of horizontal merger enhance competition in the package market, or does it reduce competition in the hospital market? The package often includes physicians and hospitals. Does this sort of vertical merger enhance competition or allow the new organization to extend market power that it formerly had only in the physician or hospital arena?

This section of the book explores these issues. In chapter 6, David Dranove discusses the changes in how health care markets should be defined. The core of his argument centers on two points. First, he argues that employers and managed-care firms increasingly purchase health care services from networks of providers. Suppose two such networks were to merge. The antitrust question is whether competition would be lessened. Typically this would be analyzed by considering the markets of each of the constituent providers in each network. If, say, two pharmacies make up one local market and each belongs to one of the merging networks, the argument would typically be that an otherwise acceptable merger must divest itself of one of these pharmacies. Dranove argues that this is the wrong unit of analysis. The nature of the new health care competition is between networks. If the networks merge, the buyers of network services face the real threat of reduced competition and higher prices. If the networks compete for the same contracts from employers and managed-care firms, in part by providing geographic coverage of pharmacies, then this sort of merger is much more likely to lessen competition than would be implied by the local market according to local market analysis. Thus the conventional approach leads to markets that are too small, focusing as they do on local providers and not areawide networks.

Second, Dranove argues that there is a market for constituent members of a network. The network seeks to include specific hospitals (or pharmacies) in its organization for purposes of having the geographic coverage that is said to be valued by employers and their workers. Here Dranove argues that the typical approach to defining the market results in too large a market definition. Typically one would use Medicare or patient origin data to examine patient flows and define the market as the geographical area in which few people leave the area to get care and few people enter it for care. Competitors are defined as all those providers within the area.

The difficulty, according to Dranove, is that while patients do travel for care they still have "option demand" for a local hospital, and they would be willing to pay something to have one available and included in their network. If so, the travel patterns do not reflect the willingness of patients to substitute a distant hospital for a local one. Dranove proposes that one might test this by examining the amount that managed-care premiums would have to drop for subscribers to willingly join a plan that excluded a local provider.

The question is obviously an empirical one, for we have no research on how much consumers are willing to pay under such circumstances. But this approach also has the potential of resulting in markets that are much too small. *Local* is undefined by Dranove, but is just one of many attributes that characterize a provider. There is option demand for tertiary services, and for particular tertiary services. There is option demand for particular styles of care: high touch as opposed to high-tech, for example, or care provided from a particular religious perspective. Operationally, the issue appears to be less one of market definition and more one of defining more precisely what the product is: aluminum foil versus plastic wrap, religious hospital versus community hospital, local provider versus distant provider. Examining the willingness to pay for the plan is a fruitful way of examining these questions. One might start, as Zwanziger and Meirowitz have done in this volume, by exploring the composition of provider networks and then moving on to exploring the effects of the composition on premiums.

Chapter 7 in this section, by Martin Gaynor and Deborah Haas-Wilson, also examines mergers in health care. Their focus, however, is on vertical combinations: arrangements between physicians and hospitals, for example, or between insurers and hospitals. Staff model HMOs are perhaps the extreme example of such arrangements. Here the insurance, inpatient, and physician service components of health care are integrated into a single firm. As table 1–2 demonstrates, other less extreme forms of organizations have developed. By late 1993 nearly 25 percent of U.S. community hospitals had entered into some form of physician-hospital organization.

The economics of vertical arrangements is complex. Analysis in the 1950s and 1960s argued that arrangements whereby an upstream firm, perhaps an insurer, acquired a downstream firm, perhaps a hospital, allowed a monopoly insurer to extend its monopoly to the hospital market by foreclosing other hospitals from access to upstream inputs. If a person wanted health insurance she had to use the hospital owned by the insurer. The logic, of course, applied to backward integration by a monopoly hospital into the insurance market, as well as forward integration by the insurer into the hospital field. During the 1970s and early 1980s the Chicago School view of vertical integration came to dominate because of a rigorous intellectual case that there was only a single monopoly profit to be had. If a firm had acquired that profit in, say, the insurance market, there was no additional monopoly rent to be had by acquiring a downstream firm. Monopolies could be extended horizontally (by acquiring other insurers, for example), but not by acquiring vertically. It follows from this logic that if vertical organizations are created or vertical exclusive arrangements are made, the effects of these must be cost reducing.

TABLE 1–2
HOSPITALS WITH PHYSICIAN ORGANIZATIONAL ARRANGEMENTS, 1993
(percent)

	Percentage of All Hospitals	Percentage of Hospitals with Arrangements
No formal arrangement	76.7	——
Physician-hospital organization[a]	15.0	64.4
Management services organization[b]	7.6	32.6
Foundation[c]	3.6	15.5
Integrated health care organization[d]	2.6	11.2

a. A joint venture between the hospital and physicians, established to own and operate ambulatory or ancillary care projects or to act as an agent for managed-care contracts.
b. A separate entity, owned by physicians or the hospitals, that contracts with solo and group practice physicians to provide administrative services, purchases physician practice assets, and acts as the agent of the hospitals and physicians in managed-care contracts.
c. A corporation, usually a hospital affiliate or subsidiary, that acquires all assets of medical group practices and negotiates or executes managed-care contracts in its own name on behalf of the hospital and physicians as a unit.
d. A parent corporation that owns and controls the hospital, a large medical group, and an insurance vehicle and facilitates the integration of contracting, operations, revenues, risk, or capital of a hospital and physician group.
SOURCE: Morrisey et al. (1996).

More recently the post-Chicago view has emerged. It argues that the single monopoly profit view rests on some very restrictive assumptions. Particularly, it requires that the upstream and downstream products are used in fixed proportions. When this assumption is removed, vertical integration may lead to higher monopoly profits or to lower costs. The answer is then always an empirical one.

Gaynor and Haas-Wilson present this economic development, apply it to the health care field, and report the results of recent antitrust cases that have sought to apply the post-Chicago view to specific circumstances. There are two key issues in all the applications. First, one of the participants must have monopoly power in either the upstream or the downstream market. Second, there must be an unwillingness of the integrated firm to sell the intermediate product to other downstream (upstream) producers.

The most-favored-nation (MFN) clause is a particularly interesting health care application of the issues of vertical integration. In an MFN contract, a hospital or other provider agrees to give the insurer or managed-care firm the lowest price it gives to anyone. From the Chicago School view such an arrangement is cost reducing: an insurer has found a mechanism that allows it to get lower prices than it otherwise would have. In return, the provider gets something of value—perhaps an assurance of predictable volume. The post-Chicago view suggests, in addition, that either of two things may be going on. On the one hand, the MFN clause may serve as a vehicle whereby the hospitals can effectively collude and prevent their neighbors from cutting prices. On the other hand, it may be a mechanism whereby a dominant insurer can delay or prevent the entry of competing managed-care plans.

The upshot of the post-Chicago view is that vertical arrangements must be considered on their individual merits. The earlier model viewed them as efficiency enhancing and, if anything, to be encouraged. In fact, there has been virtually no empirical research on the effects of vertical integration in health care. The obvious exception is the performance of HMOs relative to fee-for-service arrangements. These studies, of course, have focused on other issues, and particularly on biased selection on the part of subscribers. Given the changing nature of the health care market we need careful, rigorous investigation of whether vertical arrangements of various kinds have any effect on costs or prices.

The final chapter in the volume does provide empirical evidence with respect to mergers in the health care industry: in this case of horizontal mergers of hospitals. Robert Connor and Roger Feldman examine the effects of mergers on the prices received by rival hospitals. The basic antitrust argument is that when two or more hospitals in a market merge, it removes competitors from the market. If the remaining hospitals have more market power, prices will increase. The unique feature of the Connor-Feldman analysis is that they do not focus on the changes in the prices received by the firms pre- and postmerger. Instead, they examine the changes in prices received by their nonmerging neighbors compared with the changes in prices of hospitals in markets where mergers did not occur. The rationale is that a simple comparison of pre- and postmerger prices is subject to potential bias arising from external factors that affect the entire market. Moreover, the merger may change quality, which in turn will be reflected in the merged firm's prices. If a merger occurs in a market, however, and the merged hospital is able to raise prices, it implies that capacity has been reduced and a competitor removed. Other hospitals in the community obtain a spillover benefit; they too can raise prices. Thus, one can compare nonmerging rivals with hospitals in other markets to infer the effect of the merger on price.

Connor and Feldman examine the change in hospital operating

revenue per admission between 1986 and 1994 for more than 1,200 nonmerging hospitals located in markets in which a merger occurred and more than 2,400 hospitals in markets without mergers. They draw two conclusions. First, there was a general lack of large, statistically significant effects of mergers on the prices of rivals. For the most part, the mergers do not appear to have allowed hospitals to raise prices.

Second, the results indicate that the size of the merger matters. One can argue that simply lumping all mergers together combines large, potentially market-dominating mergers with small, innocuous ones. Connor and Feldman dealt with this by examining the changes in prices under three categories of mergers: small, medium, and large. Small mergers reflect 1–7 percent of areawide admissions. Medium mergers constituted 7–19 percent of area admissions, and large mergers had more than 19 percent of admissions. They found that small mergers had no effect on rivals' prices. The mergers were apparently too small to exert any market influence. Large mergers also failed to result in price increases; indeed prices of rivals declined. This suggests that these mergers resulted in cost savings.[2] Connor and Feldman do find evidence that middle-sized mergers resulted in higher prices for rivals. These were small in magnitude, however, averaging 3 percent.

The study suggests that the sorts of mergers that have been observed in the hospital industry over the past decade have not had significant effects on hospital prices. Given the broader issues of selective contracting and employer and provider markets examined in this book, the merger result should not be surprising. If workers, and by extension their employers, are as sensitive to the increases in premiums as the recent evidence suggests, efforts by providers to raise prices either directly to employers or to managed-care organizations will get beaten down by the very real threat that the business will go elsewhere. Mergers may have to reduce the number of providers dramatically for market power concerns to be realized.

Managed care essentially means the use of selective contracting and the arrival of payer-driven competition. This certainly implies that price has been reintroduced into the decision-making formulas of

---

2. One could make an argument that these merged hospitals were engaged in schemes of predatory pricing, lowering their prices to drive out rivals. There is little empirical evidence to suggest, however, that such strategies are successful in any industry, because the strategy typically requires the dominant firm to incur larger losses in the short run than any of its rivals, and in the long run it must be able to keep out new entrants attracted by the higher prices it hopes to charge. Moreover, I am aware of no allegations, much less any evidence, that hospitals have engaged in predatory pricing.

workers, employers, insurers, and providers. It also implies that insurance and health care markets will undergo fundamental changes. The research in this volume demonstrates that much of that market restructuring is underway. Health care markets are increasingly coming to look like other markets. There is much that is good in all this: prices are driven down to reflect true costs, and services provided come to reflect the value that consumers place on them.

This is not to suggest that there are not problems in the transition. It is not clear, for example, how much value consumers place on increments of quality, and indeed how they know quality when they see it. But markets adapt. Firms that provide quality that is too high or too low relative to consumer demands tend to be driven to the fringe; specialists emerge to provide information. In the current debate over managed-care quality it is instructive to recall what happened to the U.S. auto industry in the 1970s and 1980s. Providing inferior quality was punished in the market as new providers entered providing the price and quality mix that consumers preferred. Given the apparent responsiveness of the health care market it seems reasonable to expect as much in this market.

References

Buchmueller, Thomas C., and Paul J. Feldstein. 1996. "Consumers' Sensitivity to Health Plan Premiums: Evidence from a Natural Experiment in California." *Health Affairs* 15(1):143–50.

Center for Studying Health System Change. 1997. "Low-Cost Trends Continued in 1996." *Issue Brief* no. 10. Washington, D.C.

Dowd, Bryan, and Roger Feldman. 1994. "Premium Elasticities of Health Plan Choice." *Inquiry* 31:438–44.

Dranove, David, Mark Shanley, and William D. White. 1993. "Price and Concentration in Hospital Markets: The Switch from Patient-Driven to Payer-Driven Competition." *Journal of Law and Economics* 36(1):179–204.

Feldman, Roger, Hung-Ching Chan, John Kralewski, Bryan Dowd, and Janet Shapiro. 1990. "Effects of HMOs on the Creation of Competitive Markets for Hospital Services." *Journal of Health Economics* 9(2):207–22.

Feldman, Roger, Michael Finch, Bryan Dowd, and Steven Cassou. 1989. "The Demand for Employment-Based Health Insurance Plans." *Journal of Human Resources* 24(1):115–42.

Hillman, Alan L., W. P. Welch, and Mark V. Pauly. 1992. "Contractual Arrangements between HMOs and Primary Care Physicians: Three-Tiered HMOs and Risk Pools." *Medical Care* 30(2):136–48.

Jensen, Gail A., Michael A. Morrisey, Shannon Gaffney, and Derek K. Liston. 1997. "The Dominance of Managed Care: Insurance Trends in the 1990s." *Health Affairs* 16(1):125–38.

Jensen, Gail A., Michael A. Morrisey, and John Marcus. 1987. "Cost Sharing and the Changing Pattern of Employer-sponsored Health Insurance." *Milbank Quarterly* 65(4):521–50.

Long, Stephen H., Russell F. Settle, and Charles W. Wrightson. 1988. "Employee Premiums, Availability of Alternative Plans, and HMO Disenrollment." *Medical Care* 26(10):927–38.

Melnick, Glenn A., Jack Zwanziger, Anil Bamezai, and Robert Pattison. 1992. "The Effects of Market Structure and Bargaining Position on Hospital Prices." *Journal of Health Economics* 11(3):217–33.

Miller, Robert H., and Harold S. Luft. 1994. "Managed Care Plan Performance since 1980." *Journal of the American Medical Association* 271(19):1512–19.

Morrisey, Michael A., Jeffrey Alexander, Lawton R. Burns, and Victoria Johnson. 1996. "Managed Care and Physician/Hospital Integration." *Health Affairs* 15(4):62–73.

Prospective Payment Assessment Commission. 1996. *Medicare and the American Health Care System: Report to the Congress.* Washington, D.C., ProPAC.

Robinson, James C., and Harold S. Luft. 1985. "The Impact of Hospital Market Structure on Patient Volume, Average Length of Stay, and Cost of Care." *Journal of Health Economics* 4(4):333–57.

Starr, Paul. 1982. *The Social Transformation of American Medicine.* New York: Basic Books.

Welch, W. P. 1986. "The Elasticity of Demand for Health Maintenance Organizations." *Journal of Human Resources* 21:252–66.

Zwanziger, Jack, and Glenn A. Melnick. 1988. "The Effects of Hospital Competition and the Medicare PPS Program on Hospital Cost Behavior in California." *Journal of Health Economics* 7(4):301–20.

2
Employer Premium Contributions and Health Insurance Costs

Bryan Dowd and Roger D. Feldman

The United States relies to a greater degree than any other developed country on private sector allocation of health care resources. Despite the publicly financed Medicare, Medicaid, and Veterans Administration programs, provision of health insurance and most health care services remains largely in the realm of the private sector. Even in public insurance programs like Medicare and Medicaid, private health plans are playing an increasingly important role, with the government assuming the role of purchaser rather than provider.

Employment-based health insurance is the dominant form of coverage for the nonelderly, nonindigent population. In 1991, approximately 56 percent of all Americans received health insurance through the employment of a family member (Levit, Olin, and Letsch 1992). The health insurance offerings of employers are important in their own right because *large* employers, who are considered to offer more successful programs, have increasingly become models for public health insurance programs (Butler and Moffit 1995; Dowd, Feldman, and Christianson 1996).

Alain Enthoven (1988, 1989) popularized the concept of a "sponsor," an organization responsible for offering a choice of health plans to a defined population. Enthoven views active sponsors as an antidote to failure in the health insurance market. He writes:

This research was supported, in part, by a grant from the Robert Wood Johnson Foundation. The authors would like to thank Matthew Maciejewski for assistance with data editing and analysis, Harry Sutton for comments on the theoretical section, Colleen King and the Survey Research Center in the Division of Health Services Research and Policy, School of Public Health, University of Minnesota, for primary data collection, and the staff of the city and county governments for their willingness to complete a lengthy survey instrument. We also wish to acknowledge the helpful comments of Michael Morrisey and an anonymous referee.

Without carefully drawn rules and active management by sponsors, health plans could pursue profits or survival using competitive strategies that would destroy efficiency and equity. Individual consumers would be powerless to counteract them. (1988)

These strategies include selection of preferred risks, market segmentation, product differentiation that raises information costs, discontinuity in coverage, refusals to insure certain individuals or to cover treatment of preexisting medical conditions, biased information regarding coverage and quality, and erection of entry barriers.

One aspect of the unregulated market structure to which Enthoven objects is the tendency of employers to subsidize more costly health plans. Employers that offer a less costly managed-care plan in addition to a traditional insurance scheme, for example, often pay the premium for the managed-care plan in full, as long as it does not exceed the premium of the traditional plan. Thus, the managed-care plan has little or no incentive to improve its efficiency or to cut its price because it will not be rewarded with more consumers.

Enthoven contrasts this behavior with that of an ideal "sponsor," which would adjust its contribution so that it paid no more than the premium of the least costly plan. Employees who chose more costly plans would have to pay the extra costs with their own money. This recommendation also extends to the tax treatment of the employee premium contribution, which is often made with tax-exempt dollars. Enthoven recommends that such tax-favored "cafeteria plans" should not be allowed. Health plans would be motivated to reduce their premiums to attract more customers if these recommendations were followed.

Despite the recommendation that sponsors should set their contribution so that employees face the marginal cost of more expensive health plans, to our knowledge, only one study has tested the hypothesis that doing so will result in reduced health insurance premiums. Using data from forty-four large Twin Cities employers that offered multiple health plans in 1981 and 1982, Jensen, Feldman, and Dowd (1984) found that monthly single coverage premiums were $14 lower in firms that made a level-dollar contribution than in firms making a percentage contribution to premiums and $12 lower than in firms paying the full premium. For family coverage, the differences were $20 and $25, respectively. Analyzing the same data, Feldman, Jensen, and Dowd (1984–1985) reported that fewer than half the firms had adopted a level-dollar contribution method for the family coverage premium and only about a third paid a level-dollar contribution to the single coverage premium.

25

We know of only two national surveys of employers that have asked about the way the employer's contribution to premiums is determined. Foster-Higgins' Health Care Benefits Survey (1992) included the question, "How do you determine employee contributions from year to year for your most prevalent medical plan?" One of the responses was "employer contribution is defined and employee pays remaining amount." In 1991, 14 percent of all employers surveyed set a defined contribution. The percentage was highest among government and education employers (27 and 26 percent, respectively).

In the second survey, conducted by Lewin-VHI, Inc. (1995), governments were asked several questions about their health insurance offerings. Of the forty-five states responding to a question regarding the employer's premium contribution method, one state (Wyoming) offered only one plan. Among the remaining forty-four states, five paid a fixed amount based on the lowest-cost plan, eighteen paid some other fixed-dollar amount, thirteen paid a fixed percentage of the premium of each plan, and seven paid 100 percent of the premium.

This chapter focuses on how a national sample of large public employers managed their contributions to employees' health insurance premiums in 1994. Do these large employers follow Enthoven's recommendation to make a fixed-dollar contribution based on the premium of the lowest-cost health plan? If they do, can we detect any premium differences compared with employers that subsidize more expensive health plans on the margin? We discuss some of the conceptual issues surrounding this sponsor activity and then provide a direct empirical test of the effects of various methods of setting the sponsor's premium contribution on the average total premium (paid by both the employer and the employee).

Theory

In the market for employer-based insurance, the "sponsor" is the employer. The sponsor's job is to structure the health insurance offerings in the firm. Of particular interest in this chapter is the way in which the employer and the employees share the cost of the health insurance premium and the impact of different cost-sharing arrangements on the total premium cost.

Our theory is based on the work of Dowd and Feldman (1987), who model the objectives and constraints facing employees and employers. The employee's objective, according to Dowd and Feldman, is to maximize the utility from consuming wages and fringe benefits, including health insurance. Employees choose to work for the firm that offers the "best" (utility-maximizing) combination of wages and fringe benefits.

The employer's objective is to minimize costs, including the cost of labor. To hire labor in a competitive market, the firm's offer of wages and fringe benefits must match the offers of other firms. Thus, the firm minimizes its labor cost subject to a constraint that the worker's level of utility must be at least as high in this firm as in competing firms. Dowd and Feldman also assume that health insurance is bought in a competitive market. Finally, they assume that the firm must hire different types of workers, defined by their relative preferences for wages and health insurance. This assumption is necessary for the firm to offer multiple health plans.

It is in the employer's interest to pay as much of the employee's total compensation as possible in tax-free dollars (that is, dollars that are exempt from federal and state income taxes and FICA taxes). Generally, it is not possible for the employee's money wages to be paid in tax-free dollars, but it is possible to pay for most fringe benefits, including health insurance, with tax-free dollars. This can be done in two ways. First, the employer's share of the health insurance premium is always tax free. Second, the employer can set up "health care expense accounts" under Section 125 of the Internal Revenue Code, which allow the employee's share of the premium to be tax free.

In this simple world, the employer would pay the full premium for the health plan with the lowest amount of coverage (that is, the plan chosen by workers with a relatively strong preference for wages), and it would set up health care expense accounts to allow employees to pay for additional coverage. Employees with a relatively strong preference for fringe benefits would be able to purchase their desired level of coverage with tax-free dollars.

The real world is a bit more complex. Some employees (especially those whose total compensation is low) may prefer to take all their pay in the form of wages, and thus we observe that some firms do not offer health insurance or do not require all employees to buy it when it is offered. The firm may also not strive to eliminate employee turnover completely. Some degree of employee turnover is inevitable, and thus the employer probably tries to find the combination of wages and fringe benefits that produces the cost-minimizing amount of turnover. These qualifications to the simple model are not as important, however, as the assumption that health insurance is bought in a competitive market. As Enthoven reminds us, health insurance is not bought "off the shelf." Health plans differ in quality and coverage, including coverage of preexisting conditions. Moreover, the cost of a health plan depends on who enrolls, and this information may be available to the plan but not to the employer. In markets where the quality of products differs and where the seller has information that is not known to the buyer, it is quite likely that prices may exceed marginal costs. Therefore, part of the employer's job is to minimize the total health insurance premium by structuring its contribution so that the premium submitted by health plans equals the health plan's marginal cost.

There are several ways that the employer's premium contribution method could affect the total cost of health insurance. When the employer sets a level-dollar premium contribution no higher than the premium of the lowest-priced plan, the employee faces the cost of more expensive health plans, on the margin. Any premium contribution method that results in a higher employer contribution, with no commensurate reduction in other forms of compensation when the employee chooses a more expensive health plan, subsidizes the price of more expensive plans. Thus, employees whose employer sets a level-dollar premium contribution based on the lowest bid are likely to demand lower levels of coverage and health plan "amenities," relative to employees whose employer subsidizes the cost of higher-priced health plans. In other words, in level-dollar contribution systems, the type of health plans offered to employees *and* the distribution of employees across those plans might be different from those under a varying contribution system that subsidizes the cost of higher-priced health plans.

In addition to effects on the number and type of health plans demanded by employees and the employees' choice across plans they are offered, level-dollar contributions could contribute to lower total health insurance premiums by forcing health plans to "sharpen their pencils" and reduce their profit margins when setting their premiums. In theory, the employer could produce the same competitive pressure on health plans by forcing them to bid for entry to the firm. The fact that employees will switch health plans in response to out-of-pocket premium differentials, however, has been verified empirically (Feldman et al. 1989; Dowd and Feldman 1994–1995; Buchmueller and Feldstein 1996) whereas the *employer's* sensitivity to premium differentials across health plans, to our knowledge, has not.[1]

Competitive pressure caused by employee shopping across health plans raises the interesting issue of the tax treatment of the employee-paid portion of the premium. There are competing incentives at work regarding payment of the employee's out-of-pocket premium with tax-free dollars. On one hand, tax-free employee premium contributions

---

1. Recent studies, however, document the price sensitivity of small employers in their decision to offer insurance *at all* (Jensen and Morrisey, in this volume; Feldman et al., forthcoming).

reduce the employer's cost of compensation. On the other hand, allowing payment with tax-free dollars distorts employee choices. When employees are allowed to pay their out-of-pocket premiums with tax-free dollars under a lowest-bid level-dollar system, the effective price differential between high-cost and low-cost plans is reduced by the employee's marginal tax rate, which in turn reduces the out-of-pocket premium elasticity of health plan choice (Dowd et al. 1996). When the employee's incentive to choose lower-cost health plans is reduced, health plans have less incentive to submit premiums that equal their marginal costs.

To summarize, the simple theory predicts that the firm will pay the full cost of the low-coverage health plan. Employees will be required to pay the additional premium for higher-coverage plans. Whether they do so with tax-free or after-tax dollars depends on the relative strength of the tax subsidy versus the beneficial effects of premium competition.

Should an employer ever pay more than the premium of the lowest-coverage plan? One plausible argument in favor of varying employer premium contributions is that the premiums of high-cost health plans reflect enrollment of poorer health risks, employees with strong preferences for the additional benefits and "amenities" offered by high-cost plans, or both. Setting a higher employer premium contribution for higher-cost plans may be a way to "risk adjust" or "preference adjust" the premium for the high-cost plan. That strategy may be particularly attractive to employers when there is a strong relationship between poor risk or preference for high-amenity plans and the productivity or "value" of the employee. Older, more experienced, and more valuable workers, for example, may be in poorer health or prefer health plans with more amenities. In that situation, the employer may decide that it is less expensive to subsidize the higher-cost plan than to drop the plan and compensate former enrollees for the loss of their preferred plan.

Except for this final consideration (subsidies of higher-cost plans as a form of risk adjustment), our theory suggests that firms offering multiple health plans can minimize their total compensation costs by setting a premium contribution equal to the lowest-priced health plan. Furthermore, the theory predicts that setting a variable employer premium contribution, or allowing employees to pay out-of-pocket premiums with pretax dollars, will increase the cost of health insurance in the firm by attenuating the price competition among health plans.

Data

The unit of observation in this analysis is the employer. The population of employers for this study consisted of the governments of all cities and counties with more than 100,000 population. Public sector employers were chosen for three reasons:

• Public sector employers are more likely than private companies to offer a standard set of health plans to all employees. Benefits in private firms often vary for union and nonunion employees, salaried versus hourly employees, and other strata. In addition, private companies often have multiple establishments, each with a different set of benefits.

• In a statewide survey of Minnesota employers (Dowd, Feldman, and Klein 1987), we found that public sector employers were more likely to respond to the relatively complex survey instrument that is required to obtain the information we would be requesting.

• The Foster-Higgins survey (1992) found the proportion of employers making a level-dollar contribution to premiums was greatest in the public and educational sectors. Feldman, Jensen, and Dowd (1984–1985) also found that public employers were about 20 percent more likely than private employers to make a level-dollar premium contribution.

Data on characteristics of these employers and their employees came from a survey conducted in 1994 (Dowd, Feldman, and Maciejewski 1995). The total sample consisted of 658 city and county governments. Twenty of these were used for a pretest, and 75 did not respond to the survey, leaving 563 usable surveys (88 percent total usable response rate). Next, we dropped 81 employers that bought insurance through common purchasing pools. The purpose of this analysis was to examine the effect of employer purchasing practices on health insurance costs for employers that made autonomous decisions about health insurance, rather than turning the decisions over to a common sponsor or purchasing pool. Examples of these common sponsors, or pools, are the CALPERS program in California and the Public Employees Insurance Plan (for small local government units) in Minnesota. Of the remaining 482 employers, 164 offered a single health plan, while 318 offered multiple health plans. Our analysis focuses on employers that offer multiple health plans because the concept of a premium contribution "method" has meaning only for those employers. Making a fixed-dollar premium contribution, for example, is possible only if the employer offers at least two plans.

Several variables were difficult to obtain from the survey, especially the demographics of employees. Data on the average age of employees were missing for half the employers, and data on the average percentage female employees were missing for 28 percent. We replaced the missing data on the average age of employees, the average percentage of female employees, and the percentage of unionized employees with population means. (Only two observations had missing data on the percentage of unionization.) Twenty-eight employers had information only on their total number of employees, not the breakdown into single versus family coverage. In those cases, regression estimates of the percentage single and family were made from other variables in the model, and the total number of employees was divided among single and family coverage according to those estimates. Questions regarding the employer's contribution to premiums were asked separately for single coverage and family coverage. Respondents were also asked if they offered Section 125, which allows the employee's out-of-pocket premium to be paid with pretax dollars.

Two enrollment-weighted average premiums were calculated for each employer, one for single coverage and one for family coverage. Family coverage was defined as the policy covering the employee and an unlimited number of dependents. The weighted average premium for either single or family coverage was obtained by summing the product of the total premium for each plan times the number of employees in the plan and dividing by the total number of employees with that type of coverage. Data on market area characteristics that affect health insurance premiums came from the 1994 Area Resource File, although the actual year for individual data items varies.

An important issue in our analysis concerns the construction of variables that might be affected by the choice of premium contribution method. Two important sets of variables are the number of health plans of each type offered to employees and the coverages of those plans. Clearly, both of these variables could be influenced by the installation of a level-dollar contribution. We have data on both variables, but the issue is complicated by the fact that the coverage variables must somehow be aggregated from the health plan level to the employer level, if they are to be used in this analysis. We used the proportion of enrollees in each plan to create enrollment-weighted coverage variables. Using enrollment patterns to weight the coverage variables, however, means that these explanatory variables reflect the employees' choice of health plan, which is clearly one of the ways in which the premium contribution method can affect average health insurance costs for that employer. Thus, when the number and type of health plans and the enrollment-weighted coverage variables are included as regressors in the premium equations, the estimated effect of the premium contribution is the effect *net* of effects that work through those variables. In that sense, effects that are estimated with number and type of health plans offered to employees and enrollment-weighted coverage variables controlled are *conservative* estimates of the total effect of the premium contribution method on premiums. The estimated net effect is likely to be due to employee choice of low-cost health plans and increased competitive pressure brought to bear on health plans when they price their insurance products for that employer.

Methods

In the first part of the analysis, we present descriptive statistics on the number of government units that have adopted particular strategies for purchasing health insurance. We also compare the means of some variables for employers using different methods to set the employer's premium contribution.

The second part of the analysis consists of multivariate models in which the enrollment-weighted average health insurance premium (paid by both the employer and the employee) is regressed on a variety of explanatory variables, including the employer's premium contribution method. The basic premium regression for the ith employer can be written as:

$$PREMIUM_i = X_i \beta_x + LD_i \beta_{LD} + \sigma_u u_i$$

where: X = a vector of predetermined characteristics of the employer, employees, and market area

LD = a vector of dummy variables representing different employer premium contribution methods

β = vectors of estimated parameters

σ_u = the standard error of the estimate

u = unobserved error

A potential problem associated with estimating the premium equation is that employers are not assigned randomly to premium contribution methods. Instead, employers (and employees) choose the premium contribution method, and for that reason, there might be variables not included in our data that affect both the employer's choice of premium contribution method and the subsequent level of health insurance premiums that we observe for that employer. In that case, the relationship we observe between the premium contribution method and the health insurance costs might not be the true relationship but might be due, in part, to the spurious correlation caused by unobserved variables. Because the premium contribution method is being chosen rather than randomly assigned, econometricians refer to the premium contribution method as an *endogenous* right-hand side variable in the premium regression equation.

The most obvious potential omitted variable is the level of premiums in a previous time period. Suppose that the true relationship between contribution method and health insurance premiums is that employers who set level-dollar contributions have lower premiums. If employers with higher insurance costs in a previous period were more likely to install a level-dollar contribution *and* to have higher costs in the current time period, then the coefficient on *LD* in this example, which is expected to be negative, would be biased upward, toward zero. Suppose, however, that the omitted variable was "employees have a strong preference for higher cost health plans, and employers find it necessary to satisfy that preference." That omitted variable might be associated with a lower probability of setting a level-dollar contribution to premiums and higher insurance premiums. In that case, the effect of level-dollar contributions on premiums that we estimate would be biased downward, away from zero.

Several approaches have been suggested to deal with the effect of omitted variables. One is the *instrumental variable correction* or IV model, proposed by Heckman (1978). This method estimates an equation to predict the employer's contribution method and substitutes the *predicted* value of the contribution method into the premium equation. Because the predicted value of the premium contribution method depends only on variables included in the premium contribution method equation and not on variables omitted from that equation, the problem of omitted variable bias is eliminated. Heckman noted that the predicted value of the premium contribution method could be obtained from an ordinary least squares (OLS) equation or a probit equation. In either case, the dependent variable would equal one if the employer chose a level-dollar contribution method and zero otherwise.

A second approach to the omitted variable problem is the *sample selection model*, proposed by Heckman (1974) and Lee (1976, 1983). This approach models the joint likelihood of observing the adoption of a particular contribution method and a particular level of health insurance premiums. In our analysis, estimation of the sample selection model proceeds in the usual two-step fashion: (1) by estimating a probit equation for the premium contribution method and using the results to calculate the selectivity correction term for each observation; and (2) by including that term in a premium regression, which is estimated by OLS. In this analysis we use both the instrumental variable and the sample selection model to address the potential problems caused by employers' choosing which premium contribution method to adopt.

An important factor affecting the quality of both the IV and the sample selection estimators is the ability to identify variables that are related to choice of a premium contribution method but are uncorrelated with the error term in the estimated health insurance premium regression equation. There are several identifying variables in our data. First, we observe, at the state level, the marginal FICA and state and federal personal income tax rate for each observation. The tax rate ranges from 29 to 53 percent in our data (Lee 1995). We hypothesize that because of the theoretical interdependence of premium contribution methods and the opportunity for tax-free employee-paid premiums (under Section 125), employers in areas with higher taxes may be more likely to adopt level-dollar contributions. (We also predict that those level-dollar contributions will be accompanied by tax-free employee-paid premiums.) Because we estimate separate single and family premium equations, we can also use the contribution method for family coverage to predict the contribution method for family coverage and vice versa. This approach is made possible by the fact that the contribution methods for single and family coverage are not identical within a firm. We performed some sensitivity tests on the latter variables as instruments and report the results in the next section.

Results

The distribution of employers across the various types of premium contribution methods is shown in table 2–1. Contrary to the simple version of the theory, almost twice as many employers use some type of variable contribution method rather than a level-dollar contribution. The most popular level-dollar contribution for single coverage is to pay the premium of the lowest-cost plan. The level-dollar methods adopted for family coverage are more evenly distributed. The vast majority of firms that make variable contributions pay the full premium for single coverage. The modal variable contribution method for family coverage is a level percentage of each plan's premium.

Table 2–2 shows the relationship between contribution methods for single and family coverage. For simplicity, the contribution methods have been collapsed into four categories: (1) level-dollar based on the lowest-cost plan; (2) some other level-dollar contribution method; (3) paying the full premium; and (4) some other variable contribution method. There is a close but imperfect correspondence between contribution methods. The most striking *lack* of correspondence is for firms to base a level-dollar contribution on the lowest premium for single coverage but to adopt another method of setting the level-dollar contribution for family coverage.

In the appendix, table A–1 gives the definitions of variables used in the analysis, and table A–2 shows how the means of several variables vary across the types of contribution methods. It is important to

TABLE 2–1
EMPLOYERS' METHOD OF CONTRIBUTION
TO HEALTH INSURANCE PREMIUMS, 1994
(percent)

Method	Single Coverage		Family Coverage	
	Number	%	Number	%
Level-dollar				
Equal to premium of low-cost plan	49	15.4	28	8.8
Percentage of low-cost plan's premium	19	6.0	27	8.5
Weighted average of largest plans	7	2.2	8	2.5
Paid a level dollar, but amount is unclear	23	7.2	33	10.4
Other	15	4.7	14	4.4
Total	113	35.5	110	34.6
Other				
Employer pays				
Full premium	97	30.5	46	14.5
Full premium up to $X	4	1.3	3	0.9
Same % of premium for all plans	58	18.2	85	26.7
A varying percent of premium	29	9.1	48	15.1
Other	17	5.3	26	8.2
Total	205	64.5	208	65.4
Grand total	318	100.0	318	100.0

SOURCE: Authors.

remember that these results do not adjust for the effects of any variables. The lowest premiums for both single and family coverage are associated with a level-dollar contribution based on the lowest-priced plan. The highest single coverage premiums are found in employers that pay the full premium. Employers who use some variable contribution method other than paying the full premium pay the highest family coverage premiums.

One of the striking differences in the means of variables is the variation in the size of the government unit (number of employees) by type of contribution method. Employers basing a level-dollar contribution on the lowest premium for either single or family coverage are smaller than average, while the largest employers also set a level-dollar

35

TABLE 2–2
RELATIONSHIP BETWEEN EMPLOYERS' METHODS OF CONTRIBUTION TO
HEALTH INSURANCE FOR SINGLE AND FAMILY COVERAGE, 1994
(number of employers)

	Family Coverage				
Single Coverage	Low bid	Other level dollar	Full premium	Other variable contrib.	Total
Low bid	26	16	0	5	47
Other level dollar	1	53	1	9	63
Full premium	1	8	45	41	95
Other variable contribution	0	4	0	105	109
Total	28	81	46	160	315

SOURCE: Authors.

contribution but not one based on the lowest premium. Employers basing a level-dollar contribution to either single or family coverage on the lowest premium tend to have a higher proportion of employees in family coverage plans.

The differences in contribution methods by region are so striking that they are highlighted in table 2–3.[2] For single coverage, the South and West have above-average rates of level-dollar contributions based on the lowest-priced plan. The South has a below-average rate of full premium contributions, while the East's rate for full payment of premiums is above average. The West is below average in its use of variable contribution methods other than paying the full premium.

For family coverage, the East is below average, and the West is above average in the use of level-dollar contributions based on the lowest-priced plan. The opposite is true of full premium payment: the South is below average, and the East is far above average. The South is

2. States were assigned on the basis of U.S. Census regions as follows: South = regions 3, 5, and 7: Kentucky, Tennessee, Alabama, Mississippi, Delaware, Maryland, District of Columbia, Virginia, West Virginia, North Carolina, South Carolina, Georgia, Florida, Arkansas, Louisiana, Oklahoma, and Texas; Eastern = regions 1 and 2: Maine, New Hampshire, Vermont, Massachusetts, Rhode Island, Connecticut, New York, New Jersey, Pennsylvania; Midwest = regions 4, 6, and 8: Ohio, Indiana, Illinois, Michigan, Wisconsin, Minnesota, Iowa, Missouri, North Dakota, South Dakota, Nebraska, Kansas, Montana, Idaho, Wyoming, Colorado, New Mexico, Arizona, Utah, and Nevada; West = region 9: Washington, Oregon, California, Alaska, and Hawaii.

TABLE 2–3
EMPLOYERS' METHOD OF CONTRIBUTION TO HEALTH INSURANCE
PREMIUMS BY REGION OF THE COUNTRY, 1994
(number of employers)

| Region | Single Coverage Contribution Method | | | | |
	Lowest bid	Other level dollar	Full premium	Other variable contribution	Total
Midwest	11	21	35	36	103
Percent	10.7	20.4	34.0	35.0	100
South	22	21	23	36	102
Percent	21.6	20.6	22.5	35.3	100
East	3	8	21	24	56
Percent	5.4	14.3	37.5	42.9	100
West	11	14	16	13	54
Percent	20.4	25.9	29.6	24.1	100
Total	47	64	95	109	315
Percent	14.9	20.3	30.2	34.6	100
	Family Coverage Contribution Method				
Midwest	7	28	15	53	103
Percent	6.3	27.2	14.6	51.5	100
South	10	34	4	54	102
Percent	9.8	33.3	3.9	52.9	100
East	3	8	18	27	56
Percent	1.8	14.3	32.1	48.2	100
West	8	11	9	26	54
Percent	14.8	20.4	16.7	48.1	100
Total	28	81	46	160	315
Percent	8.9	25.7	14.6	50.8	100

SOURCE: Authors.

above average in its use of level-dollar contributions other than those based on the lowest-priced plan.

Another aspect of premium payment is the tax treatment of the employee-paid portion of the premium. On average, about three-quarters of all multiple-plan employers offer Section 125 health care expense accounts that allow employees to pay out-of-pocket premiums with pretax dollars. These accounts are found more commonly among firms that require *some* employee premium contribution. Fifty-three percent of employers paying the full premium for single coverage and 29 percent of employers paying the full family coverage premium, however, offer tax-exempt out-of-pocket premium accounts. Surprisingly, 24.4 percent of employers paying the full premium for *both* single and family coverage have set up Section 125 accounts that allow payment of employee out-of-pocket premiums with pretax dollars.

In theory, employers that pay the full premium for all plans have no reason to offer tax-exempt out-of-pocket premiums. Some employers may have misunderstood the survey question. Section 125 accounts are also used to set up flexible spending accounts (FSAs) that permit employees to pay for coinsurance, deductibles, and some uncovered medical care with pretax dollars. Some employers may have misunderstood the question about pretax payment of premiums as applying to pretax payment of cost sharing for medical care (although employers were queried separately about that aspect of Section 125 accounts).

Why do so many employers pay the full premium? Some employers may believe that subsidizing the higher-cost health plans is the only way to retain highly valued workers who are high risk or who have strong preferences for expensive health plans. Table A–2 shows the relationship between the employers' answers to the question, "Has the tendency for unequal distribution of risks caused significant problems in managing the health plans offered by the (city or county)?" and their premium contribution methods. There is no clear pattern in the data (although this result changes in the multivariate analyses). Employers who pay the full premium for single coverage are least likely to have problems with uneven risks, while employers making some other variable contribution to premiums are most likely to report problems. Perhaps the most striking result in table A–2, given the current concern over risk selection and its effects on health plan payments, is the remarkably small number of public employers who believe that uneven risk selection constitutes a problem at all.

Another possible explanation for full premium contributions is that we have misinterpreted the data. Some firms that pay the full premium may require some trade-off between health insurance and other fringe benefits, for example, through a cafeteria benefits plan. Unfortunately, our survey does not provide a definitive answer to this issue. We did, however, ask if the employer offers a financial incentive for employees to drop their health insurance. Data on the percentage of employers offering such a financial incentive by type of premium contribution method, shown in table A–2, provide no clear evidence of a systematic relationship between financial incentives and premium contribution methods.

To investigate further the determinants of the employer's premium contribution method, we estimated a probit equation in which the dependent variable was equal to one if the employer made *any* level-dollar contribution to premiums and equal to zero if the employer made any contribution to premiums that varied with the employee's choice of health plan (including paying the full premium). The results are shown in table A–3. In the multivariate analysis, employers in the western United States are more likely to adopt a level-dollar contribution method. Among the "identification" variables and "other varying contribution" are highly significant predictors. A similar probit analysis was conducted for the family coverage contribution method (results not shown). In that analysis, both "employer pays the full premium" and "other varying contribution" had negative coefficients with t-statistics larger than 6.0.

The next task was to determine whether the premium contribution method affects the average cost of health insurance paid by the employer and employee. First, we estimated separate OLS regression equations for single and family coverage in which the dependent variable was the enrollment-weighted average health insurance premium. The results are shown in tables A–4 and A–5.

We found that the residuals in the regressions were not normally distributed. That departure from normality could result in biased estimates of the statistical significance of the coefficients. To correct the skewness, we transformed the dependent variable to the natural log of average single and family coverage premiums. The coefficients on the premium contribution methods give rough estimates of the percentage change in single or family coverage premiums associated with that premium contribution method, compared with employers' contributing the amount of the lowest-priced plan.[3]

In the initial regression equations "level-dollar contribution based on the lowest bid" was the omitted reference category. Thus, the results in table A–4 indicate, for example, that average single coverage health insurance premiums were about 11.2 percent more per month for employers paying the full premium, compared with employers using a level-dollar contribution based on the lowest bid. For single coverage, payment of the full premium was the only contribution method that was statistically significantly different from a level-dollar contribution based on the lowest bid.

As discussed previously, we were concerned that some employers who said that they paid the full health insurance premium might be combining their full premium contribution with a cafeteria benefits provision that resulted in a reduction in total compensation to employ-

---

3. The precise formula for the percentage change in the dependent variable per unit change in the binary {0,1} explanatory variables is exp (β − $1/2$ variance β) −1 (Kennedy 1981).

ees who chose higher cost health plans. The result would be that employees whose employers "paid the full premium" might face financial incentives that resulted in behavior more like that of employees whose employer paid a level-dollar contribution to premiums. To test that hypothesis, we repeated the analyses using only the employers that answered no to the question, "Do you offer a financial incentive for employees to drop their health insurance?" For single coverage, the results were not substantially different. For family coverage, however, the results were different.

In the full sample of family coverage plans, the coefficients on "other level-dollar contribution," "employer pays the full premium," and "other variable contribution" were 0.051, 0.011, and 0.084, respectively. (To conserve space, the results for the full sample are not shown.) Only the coefficient on "variable contribution other than paying the full premium" was statistically significant, however ($\alpha = 0.03$).

Table A–5 shows results from the reduced sample of employers who did not offer employees financial incentives to drop health insurance. In the reduced sample, both the coefficients on "other level-dollar contribution" and "other variable contribution" are statistically significant. Average family coverage premiums for employers adopting these contribution methods are roughly 11 and 12 percent higher, respectively, than for employers setting a level-dollar contribution based on the lowest-priced plan.

As discussed in the previous section, the fact that employers are not assigned randomly to premium contribution methods creates estimation problems in our analysis. We tested for endogeneity using the Hausman test (Hausman 1978), which consists of adding the residuals from the probit regression in table A–3 to the regressions in tables A–4 and A–5 and testing for their significance. The residuals were significant in both the single and the family premium equations, indicating a level of "endogeneity" in the choice of contribution method that must be addressed in the estimation method. We tested whether the three variables representing family contribution methods were correlated with the error term in the single coverage premium equation by including those variables in one specification of the OLS equation. None of the three variables was statistically significant. We repeated the test for the family coverage premium regression and found that only the "other variable contribution method" variable was significant. Thus, we proceeded with instrumental variable and sample selection models to address the problem of endogenous choice of premium contribution method. To simplify that analysis, we aggregated the categories "level-dollar contribution based on the lowest-priced plan" and "other level-dollar contribution" into a single "level-dollar" variable.

The results in table A–6 are from premium regressions that substitute this aggregate "level-dollar" variable for the three contribution methods shown in the full regressions. These equations contain all the other explanatory variables shown in the full regression equation. In the OLS equations, the estimated coefficient of the level-dollar contribution variable was not statistically significant for either single or family coverage. The estimates from the instrumental variables and sample selection models for single coverage, however, were statistically significant, indicating a reduction in average single coverage premiums of about 7.2 percent in firms that set a level-dollar contribution. In the family premium equation, level-dollar contributions were found to be associated with premiums that were 6.1 to 5.8 percent lower than those of employers using varying contribution methods. The statistical significance of the family coverage estimates lies just outside the traditional 5 percent level. It is important to remember that these estimates, which control for the number and type of health plans offered to employees and enrollment-weighted coverage variables, are probably conservative estimates of the full effect of a level-dollar contribution method on premiums.

Discussion

We have investigated the way in which large public employers set their contribution to health insurance premiums for their employees. Simple theory predicts that employers would set a level-dollar contribution equal to the lowest-cost plan. The data do not support the simple theory. A minority of employers set level-dollar contributions of any kind, and an even smaller minority base their level-dollar contribution on the lowest-priced plan. It is true that employers who leave the employee with some out-of-pocket premium are more likely to have Section 125 plans than employers who pay the full premium, but that is not surprising. There is evidence in these data that some employers who do not set a level-dollar premium contribution may be concerned about the distribution of health risks across the plans they offer and may be using varying contributions to protect the viability of plans that attract high-risk consumers. This concern, in turn, could reflect an association between the health plan preferences of workers and their value to the firm.

Our multivariate analyses suggest that failure to set a level-dollar contribution, for any reason, carries a cost. Even after controlling for a variety of employer, employee, and market area characteristics, as well as the number and type of health plans and unobserved sources of spurious correlation, failure to pay a level-dollar contribution is estimated to increase single and family coverage premiums by roughly 7 to 8 percent.

One reason why these results are important is that they indicate that individual employers can enjoy the savings associated with setting a level-dollar contribution. It is not necessary for whole communities to adopt the strategy to bring competitive pressure to bear on health plans.

Several important questions remain, however. First, to what extent is the cost of higher-priced health plans due to self-selection of high-risk employees? Second, even if a substantial part of the higher cost *is* due to selection, are premium subsidies for those health plans an efficient way in which to compensate high-risk employees? If setting a level-dollar contribution would actually reduce health insurance costs by 7 percent, then it might be possible to pool the savings from level-dollar contributions and distribute them to what may be a fairly small number of consumers with strong preferences for high-cost plans or to put the savings toward better "carve out" coverage of high-cost cases with better disease management and possibly better health outcomes.

Presumably, employers have their own reasons for subsidizing the cost of the more expensive health plans. They may believe that the higher costs are due to self-selection of poor health risks into those plans, and they may provide the subsidy out of a sense of fairness to employees who prefer those plans. They may believe that those high-cost plans are highly valued by older, more experienced employees and that those employees would be difficult to replace if they chose another place of employment. In either case, employers are investing heavily in maintaining the financial well-being of high-cost health plans.

TABLE A–1
Variable Definitions Used in Analysis

Dependent variables[a]

Single coverage regression: Natural log of enrollment-weighted average cost of single coverage health insurance (employer and employee-paid premiums)

Family coverage regression: Enrollment-weighted average cost of family coverage health insurance (employer and employee-paid premiums)

Premium contribution methods[a]

1. Lowest-priced plan: Employer contributes the amount of the lowest-priced plan (omitted reference category)
2. "Other" level-dollar contribution: Employer pays the same amount toward the purchase of any plan, but the contribution is not the price of the lowest priced plan
3. Employer pays the full premium: Employer pays the full premium of any plan chosen by the employee
4. "Other" variable contribution method: Employer pays a different amount for different plans, but not the full premium

Level dollar: Either the first or second method, above

Employer and employee characteristics[a]

Total number of employees

Average age of the work force

% of the work force female

Employer believes uneven distribution of risk is a problem = 1 if the employer considers uneven distribution of risk across health plans to be a problem; = 0, otherwise

0–25% of employees unionized: (omitted reference category)

26–50% of employees unionized

51–75% of employees unionized

Greater than 75% of employees unionized

Located in midwestern U.S.: (omitted reference category)

Located in southern U.S. = 1 if the employer is located in the southern U.S.; = 0 otherwise

Located in eastern U.S. = 1 if the employer is located in the eastern U.S.; = 0 otherwise

Located in western U.S. = 1 if the employer is located in the western U.S.; = 0 otherwise

County (versus city) government = 1 if the employer is a county government; = 0 if the employer is a city government

(Table continues)

TABLE A–1 (continued)

Market-area variables[b]

% urban population: % of county population located in urban areas (based on 1990 Census data)

Average per capita income in county: Area Resource File (1993)

Median years of education: Median school years for persons 25 and older (1980)

Total HMOs in county (1994): Total number of HMOs in operation in the county in 1994

Hospital expenditures per capita: Area Resource File (1993)

Hospital days per capita: Area Resource File (1993)

Physicians per capita: Nonfederal, patient care physicians per capita (1994)

Marginal tax rate: Marginal FICA, state and federal income tax rates

Number and type of health plans and enrollment-weighted coverage variables

Number of fee-for-service plans offered to employees

Number of health maintenance organizations offered to employees

Number of point-of-service HMOs offered to employees

Number of preferred provider organizations offered to employees

Enrollment-weighted deductible: Enrollment-weighted average of the deductible in each health plan offered to employees

Enrollment-weighted coinsurance rate: Enrollment-weighted average coinsurance rate in each health plan offered to employees

Enrollment-weighted dental coverage: Enrollment-weighted average of a variable equal to 1 if the health plan covers dental services and equal to zero, otherwise

Enrollment-weighted mental health coverage: Enrollment-weighted average of a variable equal to 1 if the health plan covers mental health services and equal to zero, otherwise

Enrollment-weighted chiropractic coverage: Enrollment-weighted average of a variable equal to 1 if the health plan covers chiropractic coverage and equal to zero, otherwise

---

a. Employer survey data.
b. All variables except "marginal tax rate" are measured at the county level and taken from the Area Resource File. Cities covering more than one county were assigned to the county that contained most of the city's population. "Marginal tax rate" is taken from Lee (1995).
SOURCE: Authors.

TABLE A–2
MEANS OF VARIABLES IN THE ANALYSIS BY SINGLE COVERAGE PREMIUM
CONTRIBUTION AND BY FAMILY PREMIUM CONTRIBUTION METHOD

Variable	Low Bid	Other Level Dollar	Full Premium	Other Variable Contribution
Single Coverage				
Average single coverage premium, $	170.55	182.97	200.24	179.50
Total number of employees	2013.3	6141.2	2569.7	3096.1
Average age of workers	40.9	40.8	40.6	41.1
% female workers	42.6	50.0	44.9	46.5
% of employers with 26–50% of employees unionized	12.8	9.4	16.8	15.6
% of employers with 50–75% of employees unionized	19.1	18.8	11.6	22.0
% of employers with > 75% of employees unionized	23.4	35.9	38.9	27.5
% of employers believing uneven risk is a problem	6.4	6.3	5.26	12.8
% in midwestern U.S.	23.4	32.8	39.8	33.0
% in southern U.S.	46.8	32.8	24.2	33.0
% in eastern U.S.	6.4	12.5	22.1	22.0
% in western U.S.	23.4	21.9	16.8	11.9
% county governments	51.1	71.9	58.9	71.6
% offering financial incentive to drop insurance	17.0	28.1	17.9	18.3
% offering Section 125 plan	87.2	85.9	52.6	78.9
Number of FFS plans	0.6	0.5	0.6	0.7
Number of HMOs	1.6	2.0	1.7	1.9
Number of POS plans	0.2	0.2	0.1	0.2
Number of PPO plans	0.7	0.7	0.6	0.5
Enrollment-weighted % plans with dental coverage	4.3	10.9	0.2	16.5
Enrollment-weighted % plans with mental health coverage	97.9	96.9	97.9	98.2
Enrollment-weighted % plans with chiropractic coverage	72.3	71.9	81.9	72.5
Enrollment-weighted average deductible, $	65.87	59.11	77.85	91.89
Enrollment-weighted average coinsurance rate, %	4.9	3.6	3.5	4.2
Number of observations	47	64	95	109

(Table continues)

45

TABLE A–2 (continued)

Variable	Low Bid	Other Level Dollar	Full Premium	Other Variable Contribution
Family Coverage				
Average family coverage premium, $	420.07	432.11	428.32	455.74
Total number of employees	2017.1	5079.3	2394.8	3041.4
Average age of workers	41.3	40.4	40.4	41.2
% female workers	44.0	47.9	47.3	45.3
% of employers with 26–50 % of employees unionized	14.8	7.6	22.9	16.5
% of employers with 50–75 % of employees unionized	18.5	17.7	12.2	19.0
% of employers with > 75 % of employers unionized	33.3	25.3	48.8	28.5
% of employers believing uneven risk is a problem	11.1	7.6	7.3	8.9
% in midwestern U.S.	25.9	35.4	35.6	33.5
% in southern U.S.	37.0	41.8	7.3	34.2
% in eastern U.S.	11.1	10.1	34.1	17.1
% in western U.S.	25.9	12.7	22.0	15.2
% county governments	51.6	68.4	63.4	66.5
% offering financial incentive to drop insurance	22.2	22.8	24.4	17.7
% offering Section 125 plan	74.1	88.6	29.3	80.4
Number of FFS plans	0.9	0.5	0.6	0.6
Number of HMOs	1.8	1.8	1.9	1.9
Number of POS plans	0.1	0.3	0.1	0.2
Number of PPO plans	0.7	0.6	0.6	0.5
Enrollment-weighted dental coverage	7.4	10.1	12.2	15.8
Enrollment-weighted mental health coverage	92.6	100.0	95.1	97.5
Enrollment-weighted chiropractic coverage	70.4	74.7	77.6	69.6
Enrollment-weighted deductible, $	183.41	104.03	110.12	136.78
Enrollment weighted coinsurance rate, %	3.5	4.6	3.0	4.2
Number of observations	27	79	41	158

SOURCE: Authors.

TABLE A–3
PROBIT ANALYSIS SHOWING DETERMINANTS OF SINGLE COVERAGE
PREMIUM CONTRIBUTION METHOD

Variable	Coefficient	t-ratio	Prob|β|⩾0
Total number of employees (1,000)	0.047	1.506	0.132
Average age of workers	−0.029	−0.617	0.537
Percent female workers	0.012	0.889	0.374
26–50% of employees unionized	0.227	0.600	0.549
51–75% of employees unionized	0.073	0.183	0.855
Greater than 75% of employees unionized	−0.262	−0.600	0.510
Employer believes uneven distribution of risk is a problem	−1.102	−1.821	0.067
Enrollment weighted deductible	−0.002	−1.338	0.181
Enrollment weighted coinsurance rate (%)	0.015	0.403	0.687
Enrollment weighted mental health coverage	−2.019	−2.712	0.007
Enrollment weighted dental coverage	−0.419	−1.065	0.287
Enrollment weighted chiropractic coverage	−0.293	−0.991	0.321
Number of FFS plans	0.150	0.632	0.527
Number of HMOs	−0.036	−0.278	0.781
Number of POS plans	−0.127	−0.507	0.612
Number of PPO plans	0.290	1.263	0.260
% urban population	0.0005	0.038	0.969
Average per capita income in county ($1,000)	−0.022	−0.476	0.634
Median years of education in county	−0.008	−0.019	0.985
Total HMOs in county (1994)	−0.068	−1.283	0.199
Hospital expenditures per capita	−10.065	−1.224	0.213
Hospital days per capita in county	−0.313	−0.744	0.457
Physicians per capita in county	100.09	0.519	0.604
Located in southern U.S.	0.638	1.847	0.065
Located in eastern U.S.	0.232	0.434	0.664
Located in western U.S.	0.944	2.165	0.030
County (versus city) government	−0.232	−0.698	0.485
"Other" level dollar contribution (family coverage)	−0.858	−1.397	0.162

(Table continues)

TABLE A–3 (continued)

Variable	Coefficient	t-ratio	Prob|β|⩾0
Employer pays full premium (family coverage)	− 8.148	− 0.178	0.859
"Other" variable contribution (family coverage)	− 3.608	− 5.816	0.000
Marginal tax rate	2.894	1.193	0.233
Constant	4.373	0.747	0.455

NOTE: Dependent variable = 1 if employer's premium contribution is constant for all plans (LVLDOLSI = 1), = 0 if employer's premium contribution varies by health plan (LVLDOLSI = 0).
SOURCE: Authors.

TABLE A–4
SINGLE COVERAGE AVERAGE PREMIUM EQUATION

Variable	Coefficient	t-statistic	$Prob|\beta|\geqslant 0$
"Other" level dollar contribution	0.042	0.845	0.399
Employer pays full premium	0.112	2.447	0.015
"Other" variable contribution	0.032	0.713	0.476
Total number of employees (1,000)	−0.001	−0.713	0.476
Average age of workers	−0.005	−1.059	0.291
Percent female workers	−0.001	−0.686	0.494
26–50% of employees unionized	−0.035	−0.775	0.439
51–75% of employees unionized	0.014	0.317	0.752
Greater than 75 percent of employees unionized	0.052	1.196	0.233
Employer believes uneven distribution of risk is a problem	0.128	2.373	0.018
Enrollment-weighted deductible ($100)	−0.006	−0.748	0.455
Enrollment-weighted coinsurance rate (%)	−0.010	−2.933	0.004
Enrollment-weighted mental health coverage	0.126	1.238	0.217
Enrollment-weighted dental coverage	0.042	0.996	0.320
Enrollment-weighted chiropractic coverage	0.081	2.402	0.017
Number of FFS plans	0.033	1.337	0.182
Number of HMO plans	−0.009	−0.678	0.498
Number of POS plans	−0.032	−0.989	0.323
Number of PPO plans	0.022	0.947	0.344
% urban population (1,000)	0.870	0.801	0.424
Average per capita income in county ($1,000)	0.005	1.082	0.280
Median years of education in county	0.002	0.345	0.730
Total HMOs in county (1994)	0.010	1.770	0.078
Hospital expenditures per capita in county	−0.273	−0.303	0.762
Hospital days per capita in county	−0.064	−1.357	0.176
Physicians per capita in county	−0.421	−0.019	0.985
Located in southern U.S.	0.070	1.783	0.076

(Table continues)

TABLE A–4 (continued)

Variable	Coefficient	t-statistic	$Prob|\beta|\geqslant 0$
Located in eastern U.S.	0.160	3.269	0.001
Located in western U.S.	−0.003	−0.073	0.942
County (versus city) government	0.054	1.463	0.144
Constant	4.783	7.682	0.000

Ordinary least squares
Adjusted R-squared 0.159   Sample size = 318

NOTE: Dependent variable: Natural log of enrollment-weighted average single coverage health insurance premiums.
SOURCE: Authors.

TABLE A–5
FAMILY COVERAGE AVERAGE PREMIUM EQUATION

Variable	Coefficient	t-statistic	Prob|β|⩾0
"Other" level-dollar contribution	0.104	2.157	0.032
Employer pays full premium	0.029	0.530	0.596
"Other" variable contribution	0.114	2.545	0.012
Total number of enrollees (1,000)	−0.005	−3.257	0.001
Average age of workers	−0.007	−1.512	0.132
Percent female workers	−0.002	−1.856	0.065
26–50% of employees unionized	−0.044	−1.180	0.239
51–75% of employees unionized	0.011	0.287	0.775
Greater than 75% of employees unionized	0.025	0.666	0.506
Employer believes uneven distribution of risk is a problem	0.085	1.759	0.080
Enrollment-weighted coinsurance rate (%)	0.004	1.174	0.242
Enrollment-weighted deductible ($100)	−0.010	−1.417	0.158
Enrollment-weighted mental health coverage	−0.060	−0.734	0.464
Enrollment-weighted dental coverage	0.115	3.327	0.001
Enrollment-weighted chiropractic coverage	0.010	0.366	0.715
Number of FFS plans	0.056	2.674	0.008
Number of HMO plans	0.033	2.700	0.008
Number of POS plans	−0.001	−0.034	0.973
Number of PPO plans	0.043	2.065	0.040
% urban population (1,000)	−1.337	−1.497	0.136
Average per capita income in county ($1,000)	0.011	2.858	0.005
Median years of education in county	0.002	0.512	0.609
Total HMOs in county (1994)	0.002	0.392	0.695
Hospital expenditures per capita in county	0.040	0.812	0.418
Hospital days per capita in county	−0.053	−1.092	0.276
Physicians per capita in county	−8.455	−0.393	0.694
Located in southern U.S.	−0.019	−0.595	0.553

(Table continues)

TABLE A–5 (continued)

Variable	Coefficient	t-statistic	Prob|β|⩾0
Located in eastern U.S.	0.026	0.585	0.559
Located in western U.S.	−0.111	−2.674	0.008
County (versus city government	0.044	1.460	0.146
Constant	5.915	11.822	0.000

Ordinary least squares
Adjusted R-squared = 0.229
Sample size = 246 (sample limited to firms that do not have
a financial incentive for employees to drop their health
insurance)

NOTE: Dependent variable: Natural log of enrollment-weighted average family coverage health insurance premiums.
SOURCE: Authors.

TABLE A–6

COEFFICIENTS ON "LEVEL DOLLAR" CONTROLLING FOR VARIABLES
SHOWN IN TABLE A–4 AND A–5

Coverage	Level-Dollar Coefficient	t-statistic	Prob|β|⩾0	Adjusted R²
Single				
Ordinary least squares	−0.040	−1.286	0.199	0.164
Instrumental variables	−0.075	−2.055	0.040	0.160
Two-step selectivity[a]	−0.074	−2.039	0.041	0.168
Family				
Ordinary least squares	−0.025	−0.918	0.360	0.204
Instrumental variables	−0.066	−2.028	0.043	0.195
Two-step selectivity[b]	−0.060	−1.877	0.060	0.211

NOTE: "Level dollar" = 1 if the employer pays any type of level dollar contribution versus any type of contribution that varies by plan.
a. Selectivity correlation = 0.242, α = 0.087.
b. Selectivity correlation = 0.290, α = 0.071.
SOURCE: Authors.

References

Buchmueller, Thomas C., and Paul J. Feldstein. 1996. "Consumers' Sensitivity to Health Plan Premiums: Evidence from a Natural Experiment in California." *Health Affairs* 15(1):143–58.

Butler, Stuart A., and Robert E. Moffit. 1995. "The FEHBP as a Model for a New Medicare Program." *Health Affairs* 14(4):47–61.

Dowd, Bryan E., and Roger Feldman. 1987. "Voluntary Reduction in Health Insurance Coverage: A Theoretical Analysis." *Eastern Economic Journal* 33(3):215–31.

———. 1994–1995. "Premium Elasticities of Health Plan Choice." *Inquiry* 31(4):438–444.

Dowd, Bryan E., Roger Feldman, and Jon Christianson. 1996. *Competitive Pricing for Medicare*. AEI Press: Washington, D.C.

Dowd, Bryan E., Roger Feldman, and John Klein. 1987. "What Do Employers Really Want in a Health Plan." *Business and Health* 4(3):44–48.

Dowd, Bryan E., Roger Feldman, and Matthew Maciejewski. 1995. "Health Insurance Purchasing Cooperatives: Analysis of Existing Data." Final report to the Robert Wood Johnson Foundation.

Dowd, Bryan E., Roger Feldman, Matthew Maciejewski, and Mark V. Pauly. 1996. "The Effect of Internal Revenue Code Section 125 on Health Plan Choice." Mimeo, Division of Health Services Research and Policy, University of Minnesota, September.

Enthoven, Alain C. "Managed Competition: An Agenda for Action." 1988. *Health Affairs* 7(3):25–47.

Enthoven, Alain, and Richard Kronick. 1989. "A Consumer-Choice Health Plan for the 1990s." *New England Journal of Medicine* 320(1):29–37.

Feldman, Roger, Bryan E. Dowd, Scott Leitz, and Lynn A. Blewett. "The Effect of Premiums on the Small Firm's Decision to Offer Health Insurance." Forthcoming in the *Journal of Human Resources*.

Feldman, Roger, Michael Finch, Bryan E. Dowd, and Steven Cassou. 1989. "Demand for Employment-based Health Insurance Plans." *Journal of Human Resources* 24(1):115–42.

Feldman, Roger, Gail Jensen, and Bryan E. Dowd. 1984–1985. "What Are Employers Doing to Create a Competitive Market for Health Care in the Twin Cities?" *Contemporary Policy Issues* 3(2):69–88.

Foster-Higgins, Incorporated. 1992. "1992 Health Care Benefits Survey." Survey and Research Services: Foster Higgins, Incorporated. Princeton, New Jersey.

Hausman, J. A. "Specification Tests in Econometrics." 1978. *Econometrica* 46(6):1251–71.

Heckman, James J. 1974. "Shadow Prices, Market Wages, and Labor Supply." *Econometrica* 42(4):679–94.

————. 1978. "Dummy Endogenous Variables in a Simultaneous Equations System." *Econometrica* 46(6):931–59.

Jensen, Gail, Roger Feldman, and Bryan Dowd. 1984. "Corporate Benefit Policies and Health Insurance Costs." *Journal of Health Economics* 3(3):275–96.

Jensen, Gail A., and Michael A. Morrisey. 1997. "Managed Care and the Small Group Market." Chapter 3 in this volume.

Kennedy, Peter E. 1981. "Estimation with Correctly Interpreted Dummy Variables in Semilogarithmic Equations." *American Economic Review* 71(4):801.

Lee, Lung-Fei. 1976. *Estimation of Limited Dependent Variables by Two Stage Method*. Ph.D. diss., University of Rochester.

————. 1983. "Generalized Econometric Models with Selectivity." *Econometrica* 51(2):507–10.

Lee, Robert H. 1995. "State Tax Reform and State Health Insurance Reform." In *Advances in Health Economics and Health Services Research*. Vol. 15, edited by R. M. Scheffler and L. F. Rossiter. Greenwich, Conn.: JAI Press, Inc.

Levit, Katharine R., Gary L. Olin, and Suzanne W. Letsch. 1992. "American's Health Insurance Coverage." *Health Care Financing Review* 14(1):31–57.

Lewin-VHI, Inc. 1995. "The States and Private Sector: Leading Health Care Reform." Unpublished manuscript, Lewin-VHI, Inc., April.

3

Managed Care and the Small-Group Market

Gail A. Jensen and Michael A. Morrisey

The small-group insurance market has long been viewed as both conventional and problematic. The market was considered conventional in that coverage typically consisted of a single indemnity plan with reasonably large deductibles and standard coinsurance rates. Offerings of health maintenance organizations (HMOs) and preferred provider organizations (PPOs), not to mention point-of-service plans (POS), while not unheard of, were relatively rare. The category was problematic in that small employers were the least likely to provide health insurance as part of the compensation bundle paid to workers. Moreover, small firms believed that they and their workers were systematically denied coverage and subjected to long waiting periods and preexisting condition clauses.

The small-group insurance market, however, has changed dramatically during the first half of the 1990s. The proportion of small employers offering coverage has increased by more than 55 percent since its low point in 1991 to 53 percent in 1995. There has been a wholesale shift in the nature of coverage. Now two-thirds of small firms offering insurance provide coverage through a managed-care product. In many ways, this is a much more fundamental change than what has occurred in the large-group market. Unlike large employers, small employers do not offer a menu of health benefit plans. Instead, they have moved from offering a single conventional plan to offering a single managed-care plan.

In this chapter, we describe the changing nature of the health in-

Financial support was provided, in part, by a grant from the Henry J. Kaiser Family Foundation. We thank Maria Bulycheva for her able research assistance. We also thank Paul Fronstin, Catherine Hoffman, and seminar participants at the University of Alabama at Birmingham and St. Louis University for comments on an earlier draft.

surance provided by small employers. We also offer some explanations for the changes. Specifically, four features of the market help explain the growth in coverage and the shift to managed care. First, there is evidence that state-level reform of small-group insurance has both increased the probability that the smallest of firms will offer coverage and leveled the playing field for managed-care organizations. Second, our research suggests that the maturing of local managed-care markets has provided small firms with information on the nature and acceptance of managed care and resulted in an implicit certification of managed care. Third, the nature of the benefits packages, particularly in managed-care products, appears to have become more attractive of late, and thus these plans are more appealing to workers in small firms. Finally, price matters. Where the prices of managed-care products have fallen relative to conventional coverage, our findings suggest that small firms have switched to managed care.

We begin with a brief discussion of the data sources used in this study. As we discuss the trends in coverage, types of plan offerings, and improved access of both firms and their workers, we share the findings of our econometric work that seeks to explain the remarkable changes in the small-group market. Finally, we draw a number of tentative conclusions about what we may next see in the small-group market.

Data and Methods

Information on the health benefits offered by small businesses comes from two surveys that we conducted in the spring of 1993 and the spring of 1995. In both years, National Research Inc., a survey research firm in Washington, D.C., conducted telephone interviews with small businesses employing fewer than fifty workers. The sample of firms was drawn randomly from Dun and Bradstreet's list of the nation's private employers, after stratification by size, industry, and location. This list is representative of firms that have applied for a loan at some point, and on whom a credit check has been conducted. As such, it may underrepresent young firms and some small sole proprietorships (Malholtra et al. 1980). Businesses with no employees and government employers were specifically excluded from these surveys.

The two surveys used similar questionnaires and survey methods. Before each interview, the business owner was sent an invitation to participate in the study, with a time noted for the telephone interview. During the telephone survey, the interviewer asked to speak with the person most knowledgeable about the fringe benefits provided by the firm. Most often that person was the firm's owner, president, or office manager. In 1993, 1,721 small businesses were contacted, and 750 agreed to participate, and, in 1995, 1,272 were contacted, and 616 agreed to participate. These response rates of 44 and 48 percent, respectively, are typical of small business surveys.[1]

Respondents were asked whether they offered health insurance. If they did, they were then asked a series of questions about the firm's largest conventional HMO, PPO, and POS plan. If they did not, they were asked why and also about their experiences in the health insurance market. Of the 750 respondents in 1993, 495 sponsored health benefits, and, of the 616 respondents in 1995, 424 extended coverage. In both years, employees were typically offered a single plan. Altogether in 1993, 307 firms offered conventional coverage; 67, an HMO; 126, a PPO; and 32, a POS plan. The corresponding counts for 1995 were 144, 118, 129, and 76, respectively.

To produce nationally representative estimates, firms' responses are weighted by size, industry, and region in accordance with the probability of selection into the sample. In most cases, we focus on employer-based statistics, for example, the characteristics and experiences of firms purchasing insurance in the small-group market, although in some instances we present statistics on the employees who work for the firms participating in these surveys.

We also draw on data from the Health Insurance Association of America's (HIAA) Annual Employer Surveys conducted in the spring of 1989 and the spring of 1991. We restrict our focus with these data to employers other than government agencies that employed fewer than fifty workers at the time of the survey. There were 844 such firms in the 1989 survey and 1,250 in 1991. In each of these years, HIAA drew the sample of private employers from Dun and Bradstreet's nationwide list of firms, that is, the same sampling frame used for our surveys. We exploit these commonalties to examine the trend in the proportion of small firms providing coverage over the past seven years. As with our 1993 and 1995 data, we weight the firms' responses to the HIAA surveys to produce nationally representative estimates for each year that reflect the entire population of small firms with fewer than fifty employees. For more detailed information on these surveys, see Sullivan and colleagues (1990).

---

1. Our response rates are actually higher than the rates obtained in employee benefit surveys conducted by the National Federation of Independent Businesses in 1985 and 1989, which achieved 19 and 29 percent, respectively; by the Small Business Administration in 1986, 20 percent; by Roger Feldman and colleagues in 1986, 33 percent; and by Joel Cantor and colleagues in 1990, 39 percent. On these respective surveys, see Dennis (1985), Hall and Kuder (1990), ICF Incorporated (1987), Feldman et al. (1993), and Cantor et al. (1991).

In presenting findings, we highlight differences in small-firm coverage between 1993 and 1995, both in general and within types of plans. In view of the small counts for some plan types (especially in 1993), we have calculated Pearson's chi-square statistics for all comparisons made over time. In most tables, we report them directly, and, for other comparisons made in the text, we note those that are statistically significant.

The Provision of Health Benefits

We begin our analysis by examining the proportion of small firms that sponsor health benefits for their workers. Fifty-three percent of businesses with fewer than fifty employees offered health insurance in 1995 (table 3–1). Although this rate is slightly higher than in 1993 (when 51 percent offered coverage), the difference is not statistically significant.

The provision of benefits is most strongly a function of the firm's size, its incorporation status, and its age. Among firms with fewer than ten workers, half do not offer health insurance. In contrast, 86 percent of businesses with 25–49 workers provide coverage; this prevalence rate approaches that of medium-size firms. Among employers with 100–999 workers, for example, 95 percent provide health insurance (Sullivan et al. 1992). Small businesses that are incorporated are more than twice as likely as unincorporated firms to sponsor benefits (64 versus 28 percent offer coverage). Young firms are also less likely to sponsor benefits. Among businesses less than two years old, only 35 percent offer coverage, whereas among well-established firms (those in business ten years or more), 59 percent sponsor a health plan. As shown in the table, these differences by size and characteristics of firms have existed for years.

Long-Run Trends in Coverage

Table 3–1 reflects two particularly noteworthy trends. First, within nearly all categories of small firms, health insurance coverage declined between 1989 and 1991 but has increased steadily since then. In many ways, this comes as no surprise to the extent that health insurance is a normal good and that the improving economy should lead workers to buy more health insurance, leading their employers, both large and small, to offer it. Our econometric work on the decision of small employers to offer coverage over this period found that a decrease in the statewide unemployment rate led to a significant increase in the probability of coverage, even when region and year dummies were included in the model (Jensen and Morrisey 1997).

TABLE 3–1

PREVALENCE OF HEALTH BENEFITS AMONG SMALL FIRMS, 1989–1995

(percent)

Category	Firms Offering Coverage			
	1989	1991	1993	1995
All small firms	41	34	51	53
By size				
1–9 employees	32	25	44	50
10–24 employees	71	55	70	66
25–49 employees	89	77	85	86
By location				
Northeast	50	49	56	63
South	38	35	52	57
North central	37	37	46	46
West	39	27	50	46
By corporate characteristics				
Incorporated	—	50	62	64
Nonincorporated	—	17	33	28
Firm age 2 or less years	31	29	33	35
Age 3–5 years	43	27	47	41
Age 6–9 years	42	41	53	54
Age 10 or more years	40	45	57	59

NOTE: Small firms employ fewer than fifty workers. — indicates data on this item not available from the survey. Percentages may not sum to 100 because of rounding.
SOURCE: Authors' tabulations of the 1989 and 1991 HIAA Employer Surveys and the 1993 and 1995 Wayne State University Survey of Employer-Sponsored Health Benefits in Small Firms.

On first blush, this trend in the propensity of small firms to offer coverage appears inconsistent with data from the Current Population Survey (CPS) that indicate that the number (and percent) of persons without health insurance, and also the number (and percent) of workers lacking employer-sponsored coverage, have increased steadily over the period, 1989–1995. The number of nonelderly uninsured increased from 33.1 to 40.3 million between 1989 and 1995, while the percentage of the nonelderly uninsured increased from 15.3 to 17.4 percent (EBRI 1996). There need be no inconsistency, however.

First, in the fall of 1990, the economy slipped into recession, and unemployment increased. Part of the drop in employment resulted from the downsizing of firms.[2] Firms that reduced their work force showed up as smaller-sized firms in our 1993 and 1995 samples. If these companies previously offered health insurance and continued to do so after downsizing, then our estimates of the percentage of small firms offering coverage in 1993 and 1995 should be higher—and this is what we find.

Second, it is important to understand the factors underlying the trend in the CPS numbers. These are not factors that would suggest that fewer small businesses are now offering health insurance. Since 1989, total withdrawals from the labor force have become more common among the nonelderly population. Between 1989 and 1995, the percentage of individuals living in households headed by someone who did not work at all in that year increased from 10.5 to 11.3 percent (EBRI 1990, 1996). Since families without a working head have limited access to insurance, these changes in the labor market have contributed to an increase in the uninsured population.

In addition, since 1989, the composition of the labor force has shifted more toward part-time and temporary workers, who are far less likely to be eligible for employer coverage, even if the firm sponsors a plan. CPS data reflect this substitution away from full-time employment. Among the nonelderly population in families headed by a worker, 78.4 percent in 1995 were in a family headed by a full-time, full-year worker (EBRI 1996). This is down from 81.4 percent in 1989 (EBRI 1992). Because fewer workers are now eligible for employer coverage, we see an increase in both the number and percent of workers without coverage.

To summarize, employer surveys together with CPS data suggest that a larger percentage of the population now lacks employer coverage, not because employers have dropped plans, but rather because the economy and the work force have changed in ways that limit people's access to existing plans in the market. In particular, a greater proportion of Americans are simply not in the work force, and, among those who are, more are in job categories (for example, part-time and temporary) that make them ineligible for the plans that many employers are offering. These findings are consistent with recent research by Fronstin and Snider (1996) on the decline in employment-based health insurance. Although they used different methods to examine the issue, they too concluded that changes in the economy are responsible for

---

2. The downsizing of firms during recessions is well documented, although data for the most recent recession are sparse to date. For data on this phenomenon during the 1981–1982 recession, see Small Business Administration (1985).

much of the recent decrease in the proportion of the population with employer-sponsored coverage.

Table 3–1 also suggests that, although rates of coverage in 1995 still declined as firm size declined—a pattern that has always characterized provision—over time, the dispersion in coverage rates by size of firm has diminished. Compression has occurred primarily at the bottom end of the rate distribution. That is, compared with 1989, the smallest of small firms (those with one to nine employees) are now more likely to offer insurance.

Some evidence suggests that this situation is due to state reform initiatives of small-group insurance enacted over this period. Using pooled cross-sectional data on the insurance offerings of small businesses observed between 1989 and 1995, Jensen and Morrisey (1997) found that state legislation guaranteeing access to insurance plans for small firms willing to pay the market price (that is, guaranteed issue laws) caused the probability of coverage among firms with one to nine employees to increase by 0.088, or, on average, from 0.355 to 0.443. Over the period, thirty-eight states enacted reforms of this type.

A study by Buchmueller and Jensen (1997), which evaluated the effects of California's 1993 small-group reforms on the decision of such firms to purchase a plan, also found that, among firms with fewer than ten employees, coverage expanded significantly following the enactment of the reforms. Rates of coverage did not change, however, among businesses of other sizes. California's small-group reforms resemble model legislation developed by the National Association of Insurance Commissioners in 1991; many other states have patterned their reforms on the NAIC model, as well. Thus, part of the increase in the coverage rate at the lower end of the size distribution may be due to small-group reforms enacted in recent years.

Another possible explanation for this change is that Congress in 1987 began allowing sole proprietors to deduct 25 percent of employment-related health insurance premiums for the business owner and his family from the household's taxable income. Previously, owners of unincorporated businesses could not deduct these expenses. Since the tax change reduced the effective price of insurance for these individuals, coverage may have been increasing over this period among firms with this corporate status. Overwhelmingly, unincorporated firms have one to nine employees. Recent work by Monheit and Harvey (1993) supports this scenario. Using data from the 1987 National Medical Care Expenditure Survey (NMCES), they found that self-employed owners of incorporated firms had significantly higher rates of employment-related coverage than self-employed owners of unincorporated firms. If the effects of the tax change took several years to be realized—

TABLE 3–2
SMALL FIRMS' OPTIONS FOR HEALTH INSURANCE, 1993 AND 1995
(percent)

Options	1993	1995	χ^2 Statistics
Single type of health plan	78	94	46.8[a]
Choice of plan types	2	6	9.9[a]
One or more managed-care plans	22	67	189.0[a]
Only managed-care plan	19	61	170.3[a]
Conventional only	59	33	62.0[a]
HMO only	6	19	36.6[a]
PPO only	10	23	28.7[a]
POS only	4	20	58.0[a]
Two or more plans	2	6	9.9[a]
Unknown plan type(s)	20	0	

NOTE: Small firms employ fewer than fifty workers. The χ^2 statistic reflects a two-tailed test for a difference between our estimates for 1993 and 1995.
a. Significant at the 0.01 level.
SOURCE: 1993 and 1995 Wayne State University Survey of Employer-Sponsored Health Benefits in Small Firms.

and this lag seems plausible—then some of the increase in coverage among small firms may be due to it.

The Switch to Managed Care among Small Firms

Our data reveal a dramatic shift in the types of health plans offered among small firms (table 3–2). In particular, between 1993 and 1995, many small businesses began offering managed-care plans for the first time—specifically, HMOs, PPOs, and point-of-service plans. In fact, so many did so that, by 1995, managed care became the dominant form of health coverage in the small-group market, covering 70 percent of all workers insured through small firms. This figure is up from only 27 percent two years earlier. All types of managed-care plans have significantly increased their presence in the market. Between 1993 and 1995, the percentage of insured workers in small firms with HMO coverage rose from 9 to 23 percent; the percentage with PPO, from 11 to 27 percent; and the percentage with POS coverage, from 7 to 20 percent. These changes represent major new inroads into the small-group market for all three types of plans, especially for HMOs and POS plans.

The vast majority (94 percent) of small businesses that offer insurance still offer only one plan and nothing else. By 1995, however, that plan was much more likely to be a managed-care product. This fundamental change is, in many ways, more profound than the move to managed care on the part of larger employers. When large employers offer managed care, the plans are typically part of a broad menu of insurance options. Workers are free to choose among options, albeit often at differential out-of-pocket prices. In small firms, workers are offered a solo, stand-alone managed-care product whereas two years earlier they were likely to have been offered a solo indemnity plan. The sole offering has switched to managed care.

Why have small firms moved to managed care? Two recent studies, both based on the data analyzed here, shed some light on the issue. Jensen and colleagues (1997) examined the characteristics of conventional plans that were dropped between 1993 and 1995. They found that these plans differed from the population of small-firm conventional plans in two ways. First, the plans tended to have higher deductibles. The family deductible, for example, averaged $734 for dropped plans in 1993, compared with $694 among all small firms at that time. Second, most of the dropped plans had recently experienced high premium increases. Between 1992 and 1993, the dropped plans had premium increases averaging 19 percent. In contrast, the average among all conventional plans offered by small employers was only 12 percent. Managed-care plans also had smaller increases over this period, averaging between 5 and 7 percent, depending on the type of plan. This comparison suggests that the shallowness of the previous coverage coupled with rising costs may have spurred firms to switch to managed care.

Morrisey and Jensen (1997) found that differences in local market conditions also played an important role in the small-firm decision to offer a managed-care product. They hypothesized that small firms have relatively modest gains from shopping for health insurance options. But large firms offering managed care serve as a low-cost information source. Through business contacts, through their employees and their spouses, and through a myriad of other channels, small employers and their workers come to know the advantages and disadvantages of new alternative insurance plans.

In modeling the small firm's decision to offer a managed-care product, Morrisey and Jensen tested for the existence of an information spillover effect by including among the regressors the lagged market-wide enrollment shares of HMOs and PPOs in the metropolitan community in which the small firm was located. As these market shares increased, small firms were more likely to offer a managed-care plan. For each percentage point increase in the prior year's market share, the probability that a small firm would offer a managed-care product increased by approximately 1.4 percentage points. The effect was larger in 1993; a 1.0 percentage point increase then led to approximately a 2.5 percentage point increase in the likelihood that a small firm would offer managed-care coverage.

The results suggest that large firms may have been serving as informed shoppers for small firms and essentially certified the value and acceptance of managed care by adopting it themselves. In much the same way, the acknowledged shopper in an office provides information and a certification of sorts of the greatest value in VCRs or home computers. Moreover, the declining effect over time suggests that this is not an artifact of small firms being part of the managed-care market share. Rather, early diffusion likely provides information for later adopters.

The Morrisey and Jensen (1997) analysis also found that prices were key to small-firm decisions to switch from conventional coverage to HMOs, PPOs, and POS plans. Based on these data, in 1995, if the price of a managed-care plan relative to conventional coverage fell by 10 percent, then the probability that the small firm offered a managed-care plan increased by 2.4 percent. We found no statistically significant effect in 1993. Moreover, when we analyzed common reporters across both years of data, relative premium differences continued to be a key variable. Only those price differences and lagged HMO market share had a statistically significant effect on the small firm's decision to switch to managed care.

Improved Employer Access to Insurance

Access to health insurance among firms with forty-nine or fewer workers has increased since 1993. Significantly fewer small firms in 1995 reported that an inability to qualify for group coverage was a major barrier to their offering a plan or that high prices were a major barrier. Specifically, in both years we asked uninsured firms to indicate the importance that they attached to various reasons for not offering a plan. Figure 3–1 and table 3–3 summarize their responses. While, in 1993, 54 percent said that "their inability to qualify for an insurance plan at employer rates" was an important factor in not providing coverage, by 1995 only 46 percent indicated this. Significantly fewer also said that high premiums were an important reason (83 percent in 1995 as opposed to 90 percent two years earlier). While the decline in this factor is encouraging, it is important to keep in mind the general message from their 1995 responses: high prices are still the number one reason why uninsured firms do not offer coverage. Close seconds are still "uncertainty of future increases in the price of insurance," which

FIGURE 3–1
REASONS SMALL FIRMS GIVE FOR NOT OFFERING HEALTH INSURANCE, 1993 AND 1995

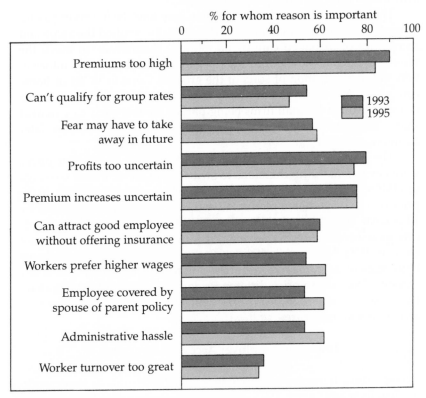

SOURCE: Authors.

75 percent told us was important, and the "uncertainty of the firm's profits," which 74 percent indicated was important. In general, the importance of different factors is not that different from what we observed in 1993. Of the ten reasons listed in figure 3–1, only the top two dropped significantly in importance; the changes observed in the others are not statistically significant.

If small employers' access has increased, albeit incrementally, why has it? Two reasons suggest themselves. First, legislation providing for state-guaranteed coverage has helped some firms that previously had difficulty qualifying for coverage. As noted, we found that firms with nine or fewer employees were more likely to offer insurance after this type of market reform (Jensen and Morrisey 1997). And most states

TABLE 3–3
PROBLEMS IN QUALIFYING FOR INSURANCE FACED BY SMALL FIRMS NOT
OFFERING HEALTH INSURANCE, 1993 AND 1995
(percent)

	1993	1995	χ^2 Statistics
Importance of "inability to qualify for an insurance contract at employer rates" as a reason for not offering health insurance			
Very important	39	37	0.2
Somewhat important	15	8	5.0[a]
Not too important	12	16	1.4
Not at all important	18	31	9.9[b]
Don't know	16	8	
For those responding "very or somewhat important," it is because . . .			
The firm is too newly established	16	14	0.1
The type of business or industry or firm makes it ineligible for coverage	14	15	0.0
One or more employees cannot qualify for insurance because of health conditions	18	26	1.7

NOTE: Small firms employ fewer than fifty workers. The χ^2 statistic reflects a two-tailed test for a difference between our estimates for 1993 and 1995.
a. Significant at the 0.05 level.
b. Significant at the 0.01 level.
SOURCE: Authors' tabulations of the 1993 and 1995 Wayne State University Survey of Employer-Sponsored Health Benefits in Small Firms.

enacted their guaranteed issue legislation in 1992 and 1993. Assuming that implementation typically took about a year, most guaranteed-coverage legislation would have taken effect in 1993 or 1994; by 1995, the early effects had been realized. These measures may well have done what they were intended to do: reduce instances of firms being told they do not qualify for coverage.

A second reason is that the growing presence of HMOs in the small-group market has made coverage available to firms that had experienced access problems. Under the 1973 HMO act, guaranteed coverage and renewal are a requirement for federally qualified plans, and such plans account for most HMO enrollment in the United States. If federally qualified HMOs have begun vigorously marketing to small firms, businesses that have been turned down by other insurers stand to gain because these HMOs are obligated to take all comers.

Changes in marketing by HMOs could be an indirect consequence of the states' reform legislation for small-group insurance. As Buchmueller and Jensen (1997) have noted, for many leading HMOs, small-group reform has not required major changes in the way that they do business. Rather, such reform has served to outlaw practices used by some of their indemnity competitors, such as redlining, which has been documented in the small-group market (McLaughlin and Zellers 1994). In essence, small-group reform may have helped to level the playing field so that nonindemnity insurers can now compete without fear of adverse selection against their plans. Indeed, some case studies on the effects of small-group initiatives in various states have documented that, following reform, the affected markets experienced an exit of small indemnity insurers and the entry of HMOs (Chollet and Paul 1994; Markus et al. 1995). The timing of the HMOs' entry into these local markets is clearly consistent with this hypothesis, namely, that small-group reform has enabled managed-care plans to come in and compete under now-parallel terms of issue and thereby limit potential adverse selection against their plans.

Simply enabling market entry and assuring a level playing field, however, could not have generated small firms' obvious demand for managed care, in and of itself. Rather, large-firm certification and the price of coverage were key. As noted, our data suggest that firms that began offering managed care did so because the price of these plans relative to conventional coverage fell in their local market (Morrisey and Jensen 1997). We did not find that their decisions depended on the presence of small-group reform per se. Thus, while small-group reform may have been necessary to bring about the changes in the market—by setting the stage for entry and new competition—it was not sufficient to cause firms to switch plans. Small firms moved only after a better deal came their way.

Improved Worker Access to Insurance in Small Firms That Offer Coverage

Other dimensions of access to insurance concern which workers within a firm are eligible to participate in an employer's plan when one is offered and, also, how long they must wait to have their medical expenses covered by the plan, assuming they can participate in it. Historically, small firms have been less likely to include part-time workers in their plans and less likely to include retirees, compared with larger

TABLE 3–4
EXCLUSION OF WORKERS OR DEPENDENTS FROM HEALTH PLANS
BECAUSE OF POOR HEALTH AMONG SMALL FIRMS, 1993 AND 1995
(percent)

	1993	1995	χ^2 Statistics
Conventional plans			
Yes	9	4	3.6[a]
No	91	96	3.6[a]
Don't know	0	0	
HMO plans			
Yes	1	0	1.2
No	98	99	0.3
Don't know	1	1	
PPO plans			
Yes	5	4	0.1
No	95	96	0.1
Don't know	0	0	
POS plans			
Yes	6	1	2.3
No	93	99	3.0[a]
Don't know	2	0	

NOTE: Small firms employ fewer than fifty workers. The χ^2 statistic reflects a two-tailed test for a difference between our estimates for 1993 and 1995.
a. Significant at the 0.10 level.
SOURCE: Authors' tabulations of the 1993 and 1995 Wayne State University Survey of Employer-Sponsored Health Benefits in Small Firms.

firms. There has also been concern that their plans' clauses about pre-existing conditions were inferior to those typically offered by large firms. That great concern, in fact, prompted most states to set specific standards for these provisions as part of small-group reform initiatives.

Among small firms that offer health insurance, our data suggest that worker access to benefits has increased in four ways since 1993. First, there are significantly fewer instances of particular workers or dependents being excluded from a plan because of poor health. In both surveys, we asked small firms offering coverage whether any workers or dependents were excluded from a plan because of health conditions and, if so, which plans they were excluded from. As table 3–4 indicates, between 1993 and 1995, significantly fewer firms indicated that some individuals were being singled out for exclusion from conventional plans or point-of-service plans. While the data suggest that there may also have been a decline in exclusions from PPOs and HMOs, the changes actually observed were not large enough to be statistically significant.

Second, the categories of workers eligible to participate in employer plans are broader. Table 3–5 shows that significantly more small firms are covering part-time workers under their plans. The increase between 1993 and 1995 was substantial. Whereas only one of every five small firms covered part-time employees in 1993, by 1995 one of every three covered such workers.

Third, waiting periods to enroll after being hired shortened between 1993 and 1995 (table 3–5), with more workers being covered within three months of hire.

Finally, the preexisting condition clauses in small-group plans have become less stringent over time, so more medical conditions are being covered sooner than they otherwise would be. More workers have plans with no restrictions or limits on preexisting conditions. This is due to two trends. First, and perhaps more obvious, many more workers are in HMOs, which (with rare exception) do not impose preexisting condition clauses. The second reason is that non-HMO plans substantially relaxed their clauses between 1993 and 1995 (table 3–5). One explanation is that they did so in response to increased competition from HMOs, which, even in the small-group market, tend to cover preexisting conditions immediately without a wait. We do not think that these changes are due to the recent state standards for these clauses. As our earlier work shows, most small-group plans already met the standards, so the regulations should have been nonbinding (Morrisey et al. 1994).

Changes in Employee Cost Sharing

Small businesses have also made changes in their workers' cost-sharing provisions since 1993. Significantly fewer workers are being asked to contribute toward premiums (table 3–6). In 1995, only 30 percent of workers were required to contribute toward individual premiums, which is down from about half of insured workers (49 percent) in 1993. Forty-six percent were required to contribute toward family premiums, which also is down from 59 percent two years earlier. The average percent contribution among those required to contribute, however, rose over the period, from 39 to 44 percent for individual coverage and from 47 to 54 percent for family coverage. Both represent significant increases.

In making the switch to a managed-care plan, some firms that

TABLE 3–5

ELIGIBILITY AND WAITING PERIODS FOR PLAN ENROLLMENT AND
PREEXISTING CONDITION CLAUSES AMONG SMALL FIRMS PROVIDING
INSURANCE, 1993 AND 1995

(percent)

	1993	1995	χ^2 Statistics
Eligible to participate in health plan			
Employees' family members	85	87	1.1
Part-time employees	19	32	21.2[a]
Retired employees	19	19	0.0
Owner (or owners) of firm	80	82	0.8
Waiting period until enrollment from time of hire for a full-time employee			
Immediately enrolled	20	21	0.1
1–3-month wait	54	63	7.6[a]
4–9-month wait	9	8	0.3
12 months or longer	5	6	0.4
Unknown	13	2	
Preexisting condition clauses			
Conventional plans			
No restrictions or limits	30	37	2.1
1–5-month wait	3	3	0.0
6–12-month wait	24	33	4.3[b]
More than 12 month wait	3	5	0.9
Other/missing	40	22	
PPO plans			
No restrictions or limits	15	28	6.8[a]
1–5-month wait	11	4	5.4[b]
6–12-month wait	46	48	0.1
More than 12 month wait	4	0	0.0
Other/missing	25	20	
POS plans			
No restrictions or limits	14	30	3.2[c]
1–5-month wait	2	5	0.5
6–12-month wait	52	31	4.5[b]
More than 12 month wait	0	4	1.3
Other/missing	32	30	

NOTE: Small firms employ fewer than fifty workers. The χ^2 statistic reflects a two-tailed test for a difference between our estimates for 1993 and 1995.
a. Significant at the 0.01 level.
b. Significant at the 0.05 level.
c. Significant at the 0.10 level.
SOURCE: Authors' tabulations of the 1993 and 1995 Wayne State University Survey of Employer-Sponsored Health Benefits in Small Firms.

TABLE 3–6
PREMIUM SHARING FOR EMPLOYER-SPONSORED HEALTH INSURANCE
IN SMALL FIRMS, 1993 AND 1995
(percent)

	1993	1995	χ^2 Statistics
Single coverage			
Workers required to contribute toward premium			
Yes	49	30	33.9[a]
No	41	55	19.3[a]
Don't know/missing	10	15	
Average contribution toward premium			
Across all plans	39	44	2.8[b]
By type of plan			
Conventional	39	54	9.0[a]
HMO	35	42	0.8
PPO	39	38	0.0
POS	—	37	
Family coverage			
Workers required to contribute toward family coverage premium			
Yes	59	46	14.3[a]
No	29	28	0.2
Don't know/missing	13	26	
Average contribution toward premium			
Across all plans	47	54	4.5[c]
By type of plan			
Conventional	46	57	4.8[c]
HMO	46	54	1.2
PPO	55	57	0.9
POS	46	46	0.0

NOTE: Small firms employ fewer than fifty workers. Data reflect the population of insured workers. The χ^2 statistic reflects a two-tailed test for a difference between our estimates for 1993 and 1995.
a. Significant at the 0.01 level.
b. Significant at the 0.10 level.
c. Significant at the 0.05 level.
SOURCE: Authors' tabulations of the 1993 and 1995 Wayne State University Survey of Employer-Sponsored Health Benefits in Small Firms.

switched may have dropped their premium contribution requirements for workers. Among small firms in 1995, managed-care premiums were, in fact, lower than those for conventional coverage. Thus, the premium savings from the switch may have been passed on to workers by changing from a required contribution to a full-payment arrangement, especially when the required contribution was fairly small to begin with. If this happened, the average percentage of contributions among those workers required to contribute would have likely risen; table 3–6 reflects this situation. This switch is also certainly consistent with the strong economy in the mid-1990s and with the relatively slow rise in wages.

Deductibles for conventional plans in small firms have actually fallen as a result of the shift to managed care (table 3–7). As noted, many conventional plans that small firms dropped had higher-than-average deductibles, and those plans that were not dropped had lower-than-average deductibles. As a result, the average has declined slightly, from $329 to $305 per individual and from $716 to $708 per family. While still much larger than those found in conventional plans of large firms, the gap by size of firm has narrowed since 1993.

At the same time, copayments for HMO plans have risen significantly. Copayments of $10–20 per visit are now the norm, instead of $3–9 per visit in 1993. As with conventional coverage, HMO coverage for small firms is not as generous as in large firms, although the differences between the two are not that large. They differ primarily in that copayments per visit are higher in the plans in small firms.

Discussion

Four major conclusions emerge from this analysis. First, more small firms are offering coverage now than in the late 1980s. From our analysis, it is clear that much of this has been driven by the aggregate U.S. economy. Growth in the economy does increase the probability that a small firm will offer health insurance benefits. Thus, "it's the economy, stupid" applies in health insurance as it does in so many areas.

We measured growth in terms of the local unemployment rate. Less unemployment was associated with higher probabilities of coverage. This suggests that the imminent retirement of the baby-boom generation will increase the proportion of the work force with employer-sponsored coverage. The retirees will have relatively high incomes and can be expected to continue to demand goods, and services. Their withdrawal from the labor force, however, will increase the demand for remaining workers, push up compensation, and disproportionately in-

TABLE 3–7
Cost Sharing at the Point of Purchase in Small Firms,
1993 and 1995
(dollars and percent)

	1993	1995	t-Statistics χ^2 Statistics
Average annual deductibles ($)			
Conventional			
Single	329	305	32.4[a]
Family	716	708	92.4[a]
PPO			
In-plan	266	280	3.3[b]
Out-of-plan	1,072	386	161.8[a]
Point-of-Service			
In-plan	–	218	
Out-of-plan	261	314	9.5[a]
HMO copayments (%)			
Percentage of workers facing copayment per visit			
None	18	8	4.4[b]
$2 or less	—	2	
$3–9	32	18	6.8[a]
$10–20	3	67	32.8[a]
Other/don't know	23	7	

Note: Small firms employ fewer than fifty workers. Data reflect the population of insured workers. The χ^2 statistic reflects a two-tailed test for a difference between our estimates for 1993 and 1995.
a. Significant at the 0.01 level.
b. Significant at the 0.05 level.
Source: Authors' tabulations of the 1993 and 1995 Wayne State University Survey of Employer-Sponsored Health Benefits in Small Firms.

crease the probability that workers will have coverage through their workplace.

Growth is not a short-run solution to the problem of the uninsured, however. Our data, when compared with the CPS data on coverage held by individuals, suggest that much job growth in the mid-1990s has been of the part-time variety and not typically of the sort that carries health insurance coverage. Further, withdrawal from the labor force by the head of household often brings with it the loss of

73

health insurance for other members of the family. If society wishes to expand coverage more quickly, other efforts will be necessary.

Second, state laws dealing with insurance underwriting have increased the likelihood that the smallest of small firms will offer coverage. This increase appears to come primarily from laws dealing with the guaranteed issuance of coverage. Moreover, as we look across the range of studies, it appears that the reforms have helped set the stage for managed care. While not directly prompting firms to shift coverage, the laws may have leveled the playing field, particularly for HMOs. In addition to providing for guaranteed issuance of coverage, the laws typically limited waiting periods for coverage and defined and limited limitations for preexisting condition. HMOs were much less likely to use provisions, in part because of the terms of the 1973 federal HMO act.

The state reforms have been widespread. Some forty-five states have enacted laws dealing with preexisting conditions, for example. Our review suggests that these laws have had only a modest effect on the provision of health insurance. Thus, we doubt that the recently enacted Health Insurance Portability Act will have much of an impact on small employers and their workers. As applied to small employers, the law largely follows existing state actions, and the state laws have already made what little impact could have been expected.

Third, large employers play a two-pronged role in the managed-care market. They are well known as the engine of managed-care growth over the 1980s and 1990s. Analysts have suggested that managed-care growth in some regions of the country will be limited by the absence of many large employers.

Our analysis suggests that this may be too narrow a view. It appears that adoption of managed care by large employers serves as an information and certification vehicle for smaller firms. Thus, managed care may indeed grow significantly in areas dominated by small employers once the larger employers in the area come to offer HMOs, PPOs, and POS plans. In this special sense, managed care does not appear limited by the market.

Finally, price matters. It matters in two dimensions. First, the move to managed care, in part, has been motivated by the relatively lower premiums offered by managed-care firms. To the extent that relative prices continue to be lower (or to fall more), managed-care penetration in the small-group market is likely to remain high and to grow further.

More fundamentally, however, the key to the provision of health insurance continues to be price. Our survey data of small employers continue to find that price is paramount to offering coverage. If workers (and their employers) are to buy coverage, prices must fall. Our data, however, indicate that, while the rates of increase in health insurance premiums have declined since 1989, they have nonetheless increased. Only since 1995 have the rates of premium increase been below the level of general inflation. If substantially more workers in small firms are to buy health insurance, this one-time observation of lower real prices must become a trend. Indeed, we see market forces and the potential decrease in health insurance premiums as the most promising element on the horizon to expand health insurance coverage among workers in small firms.

References

Buchmueller, Thomas C., and Gail A. Jensen. 1997. "Small Group Reform in a Competitive Managed Care Market: The Case of California, 1993 to 1995." *Inquiry* 34(3).

Cantor, Joel, et al. 1991. "Business Leaders' Views on American Health Care." *Health Affairs* 10: 98–105.

Chollet, Deborah J., and Rebecca R. Paul. 1994. "Community Rating: Issues and Experience." Working paper. Alpha Center, Washington, D.C., December.

Dennis, William J., Jr. 1985. *Small Business Employee Benefits*. Washington, D.C.: National Federation of Independent Business.

Employee Benefit Research Institute. 1990. "Uninsured in the United States (Analysis of the March 1990 Current Population Survey)." EBRI Special Report 8. Washington, D.C.: EBRI, September.

——. 1992. "Sources of Health Insurance and Characteristics of the Uninsured (Analysis of the March 1991 Current Population Survey)." EBRI Special Report 14. Washington, D.C.: EBRI, February.

——. 1996. "Sources of Health Insurance and Characteristics of the Uninsured (Analysis of the March 1996 Current Population Survey)." EBRI Issue Brief 179. Washington, D.C.: EBRI, November.

Feldman, Roger, et al. 1993. "The Effect of HMOs on Premiums in Employment-based Health Plans." *Health Services Research* 27: 779–812.

Fronstin, Paul, and Sarah C. Snider. 1996. "An Examination of the Decline in Employment-based Health Insurance between 1988 and 1993." *Inquiry* 33: 317–25.

Hall, Charles, and J. Kuder. 1990. *Small Business and Health Care: Results of a Survey*. Washington, D.C.: National Federation of Independent Business Foundation.

ICF Incorporated. 1987. *Health Care Coverage and Costs in Small and Large Businesses*. Final report prepared for the U.S. Small Business Administration. Washington, D.C.: ICF.

Jensen, Gail A., and Michael A. Morrisey. 1997. "Small Group Reform and Insurance Provision by Small Firms, 1989–1995." Working paper. Institute of Gerontology, Wayne State University, Detroit, August.

Jensen, Gail A., Michael A. Morrisey, Shannon Gaffney, and Derek K. Liston. 1997. "The New Dominance of Managed Care: Insurance Trends in the 1990s." *Health Affairs* 17: 125–36.

Malholtra, Suresh, Kenneth M. McCaffree, John M. Wills, and Jean Baker. 1980. *Employment Related Health Benefits in Private Nonfarm Business Establishments in the United States. Vol. 2. Sampling and Survey Strategy.* Final report prepared for the Department of Labor. Seattle: Battelle Human Affairs Research Centers.

Markus, Anne R., Kala Ladenheim, and Lisa Atchison. 1995. "Small Group Market Reforms: A Snapshot of States' Experiences." Special report prepared for the Commonwealth Fund, New York, February.

McLaughlin, Catherine G., and Wendy K. Zellers. 1994. *Small Business and Health Care Reform.* School of Public Health, University of Michigan, Ann Arbor.

Monheit, Alan C., and P. Holly Harvey. 1993. "Sources of Health Insurance for the Self-Employed: Does Differential Taxation Make a Difference?" *Inquiry* 30: 293–305.

Morrisey, Michael A., and Gail A. Jensen. 1997. "Switching to Managed Care in the Small Employer Market." *Inquiry* 34(3).

Morrisey, Michael A., Gail A. Jensen, and Robert J. Morlock. 1994. "Small Employers and the Health Insurance Market." *Health Affairs* 13:149–61.

Small Business Administration. 1985. *The State of Small Business, 1985.* Washington, D.C.: U.S. Government Printing Office.

Sullivan, Cynthia B., et al. 1990. *Technical Methodology: HIAA Survey of Employer-sponsored Health Benefit Plans.* Washington, D.C.: Health Insurance Association of America, February.

———. 1992. "Employer-sponsored Health Insurance in 1991." *Health Affairs* 12: 172–85.

4

Strategic Factors in Hospital Selection for HMO and PPO Networks

Jack Zwanziger and Adam Meirowitz

Even without passage of comprehensive health reform, the health care system is undergoing a fundamental restructuring. Market forces and managed care are at the core of this transformation. Almost three-quarters of U.S. workers with health insurance are insured through either health maintenance organizations (HMOs), point-of-service plans (POS), or preferred provider organizations (PPOs) (Jensen et al. 1997). Enrollment in these plans is expected to increase as these plans expand into the publicly financed sector. More than twenty states have applied for waivers from the Health Care Financing Administration (HCFA) to enroll Medicaid recipients in managed-care plans, while federal policy makers consider strategies to spur growth in Medicare HMO enrollment. Managed care has not only grown but changed: an evolution in the organizational structure of managed-care firms and in their contractual relationships with providers has taken place. Today's HMO is far different from its early predecessors both in structure and in its effect on its market.

An important aspect of these plans is that they contract with a subset of the providers in the areas they serve. While the network managers for individual plans are attempting to improve the market position of their plan, the cumulative effect of their individual decisions could restructure the health care system. As managed care becomes a dominant mode of insurance, hospitals with characteristics that managed-care plans tend to favor will survive; those lacking such characteristics will be forced to close, merge, or change.

This study uses a unique, internally developed, managed-care plan–hospital contracting database. We used the data to study the factors that influence the contracting decision between managed-care plans (HMOs and PPOs) and general acute care hospitals in a sample of fourteen large standard metropolitan statistical areas (SMSAs) conducted in 1993.

We used multivariate regressions to identify the hospital, plan, and SMSA characteristics that influence the probability of a contract between the plan and the hospital. The plan characteristics include type of plan (HMO or PPO; the HMO category may be further subdivided), ownership, size, multilocality (yes or no), and age. Hospital characteristics include size, ownership, location (city, suburbs), teaching status, its relative costliness ([operating expenses/adjusted discharge]/the SMSA average), and the financial pressure exerted on the hospital by Medicare and Medicaid. The primary SMSA characteristics of interest include the penetration and rate of growth of managed-care plans.

The specific hypotheses that motivated our analysis include the following:

• Publicly owned hospitals are less likely to receive contracts reflecting the preferences of working- and middle-class subscribers.

• Larger hospitals are more likely to receive contracts reflecting plan preferences for more comprehensive service breadth.

• Low-cost hospitals, relative to the hospitals within the SMSA, are more likely to contract than higher-cost hospitals. Of utmost importance to a managed-care plan is the cost of care at a particular hospital. Managed-care plans will exclude a hospital from its provider network if the hospital cannot deliver the services at a reasonable cost.

• Established plans are likely to have smaller hospital networks.

Background

With the failure of Congress to adopt a national health care reform package, public and private sector policy makers are continuing to search for mechanisms to control health care expenditures. One such mechanism is managed care. The growth of managed-care plans over the past decade is leading to a radically restructured health care marketplace. In the early 1980s, less than 20 percent of the insured population was enrolled in such plans, and most of these were in Kaiser-model HMOs where the HMO owned the hospitals its members used. With the passage of selective contracting laws, first in California and then in other states, health insurers had greater flexibility to develop alternative health plans and to test different design features. This increased competition in the insurance market led to a burst of innovation and a proliferation of choices available to consumers. PPOs, for example, grew rapidly by offering a wide choice of providers (we use the term *provider* to refer to both physicians and hospitals) in their networks, combined with lower monthly premiums (compared with prevailing indemnity plans), and financial incentives to use network providers, while still providing some financial coverage for out-of-network utilization (unlike HMOs). The number of people voluntarily selecting these plans grew dramatically.

At the same time, innovations were being introduced in the HMO market. The new HMOs differed from closed-system HMOs (such as Kaiser) in ways that made them attractive to both providers and consumers. Physicians could join the HMOs either as individuals or as part of an independent practice association (IPA) or in a group practice, while hospitals could contract with the plans on a selective basis. Consumers had a wide choice of private providers in these plans, and the monthly premiums were generally less than conventional indemnity plans. During this same time period, employers began changing their contribution rates to health insurance plans, requiring employees to pay a larger share if they selected plans with higher premiums.

The response of consumers and providers to these changes has been nothing short of remarkable. Sixty-five percent of workers at medium and large companies are enrolled in managed-care plans (Eckholm 1994). This growth has continued. By 1995, Jensen et al. (1997) found that 75 percent of insured employees had enrolled in managed-care plans. Providers are increasingly affiliating with these plans (three-fourths of all physicians contract with managed-care plans), and revenue from managed-care plans accounts for an increasing proportion of physician income (Simon and Born 1996). The proliferation of managed care is continuing to shape the health care industry as insurers and providers vie to strengthen their bargaining positions. HMOs are increasingly consolidating through mergers and buyouts. Physicians and hospitals have begun to affiliate as well to build large organizations capable of exerting countervailing market power. Mergers in the health sector exceeded the value of mergers in any other industry in 1994 (Securities Data Company 1994).

Nationally, we know very little about the effects of these changes in the health services market. Information about the effects of market structure is also critical for the federal agencies and state attorney general offices struggling to define criteria for challenging mergers on the basis of antitrust doctrine.

To assess system performance fully, we must capture the interdependencies of provider and insurer markets. To date, studies of the determinants of hospital costs have focused principally on hospital market structure as a driving force. Similarly, studies of health insurance premiums have included measures of either hospital market structure or plan competition, but very few have included both. Failure to integrate the dynamics of these markets has led to seemingly conflicting results. The impact of hospital competition, for example, depends on the structure of the insurance market, particularly the size and sophistication of the managed-care sector. Previous studies of hospital competition and its effect on hospital costs have shown that before the growth of managed-care programs, more competitive markets had higher hospital costs (Joskow 1980; Wilson and Jadlow 1982; Luft and Maerki 1984–1985; Farley 1985; Robinson and Luft 1985; and Luft et al. 1986). Under cost-based, fee-for-service systems, providers competed on the basis of services and quality, rather than price, leading to higher costs in more competitive markets. More recent research on hospital competition suggests that competition in hospital markets can lead to efficiencies when the insurance market includes sufficient managed-care penetration (Melnick and Zwanziger 1988; Zwanziger and Melnick 1988; Melnick et al. 1992; Robinson 1991; Chernew 1993; Feldman and Dowd 1986; and McLaughlin 1988). Other studies, however, such as a recent one by Gruber (1994), show no effect.

Few studies directly address the factors underlying provider contracting. Johns, Derzon, and Anderson (1985) and Brown, Cousineau, and Price (1985) described the initial factors that led to securing a contract with the California MediCal (Medicaid) program after it began to contract with a selected subset of hospitals. They showed that high MediCal volume was an important predictor of success. A statistical analysis by Mennemeyer and Olinger (1989) confirmed this finding. Both Johns (1989) and Melnick, Zwanziger, and Verity-Guerra (1989) showed that selective contracting was succeeding in reducing hospital costs. Several studies focused on the contracting process. Melnick et al. (1992) studied the prices negotiated by hospitals with a large California PPO. They found a distinct pricing pattern with hospital costs, the competitiveness of the hospital market, and other measures of relative bargaining power as predicting the contracting price.

The most comprehensive analysis to date of the factors influencing hospital contracting was conducted by Feldman et al. (1990). They studied six HMOs in four unnamed markets and found that IPA-model HMOs appeared to be relatively unsystematic in their contracting decisions, whereas staff-network model HMOs used quality "markers," such as the presence of residency programs (positive) and public ownership (negative) in making a contracting decision. In addition, they found that although cost did not appear to be a factor in the contracting decision, plans were successful in steering beneficiaries to lower-priced hospitals.

No study has examined all the factors that lead to a hospital's inclusion in a managed-care plan's network for a large sample of managed-care plans. As these plans become the dominant form of insurance, especially as more Medicare beneficiaries join HMOs, a hospital's survival will depend on competing successfully in this arena. This study is the first to analyze these factors for a national sample of SMSAs, a variety of managed-care plans, and a large and diverse population of hospitals.

Data and Methods

Data Collection. We have selected a sample of thirteen large SMSAs from SMSAs with 1990 populations of more than 1 million and substantial managed-care penetration in 1992. We then selected approximately ten of the largest HMOs and PPOs with service areas covering the SMSA. We contacted each plan by telephone. When we reached the appropriate person, we requested the list of hospitals in their plan's hospital network. If asked, we sent a confirming letter to show that ours was indeed a legitimate research project, rather than one with a marketing or consulting objective. In our experience, fewer than 5 percent of plans contacted refused to provide us with the list of hospitals in their network. Once we received the hospital list, we entered it in a hospital-plan spreadsheet for that SMSA. These data sets included hospital and plan names and other identifying information together with an indicator of whether that specific plan had a contract with a given hospital in that SMSA. The hospital was manually linked to the hospital identifier in the American Hospital Association (AHA) identifier and the plan to the plan identifier in the SMG Marketing Group 1992 Annual Survey of HMOs and PPOs.

Estimating the Probability of a Contract. We model the probability of a contract between a managed-care plan and a hospital using multivariate logistic regression. For hospital i and plan j,

$$Prob \text{ (Contract}_{ij}) = f(PCHAR_j\ HCHAR_i) + e_{ij} \qquad (4\text{--}1)$$

where

$PCHAR_j$ is a vector of plan characteristics,
$HCHAR_i$ is a vector of hospital characteristics,
e_{ij} is white noise.

We estimated three distinct models. The first assumed no correlation in errors justifying a simple logistic model, the second and third assumed that there were constant SMSA- and plan-level factors, respectively, that influenced the probability of a contract and used a fixed effect (*FE*) approach to incorporating them in the model. For the SMSA-level *FE* model, we add dummy variables for twelve of the thirteen SMSAs in the data set to the plans and hospital variables in the initial model. For the plan-level *FE* model, we add dummy variables for 134 of the 135 plans included in the data set to the hospital variable in the initial model.

The unit of analysis is a dyadic pairing of hospitals and plans. The dependent variable of interest is the existence of a contract (inclusion of the hospital in the plan's selective contracting network). Measures of hospital size, costliness, and involvement in teaching (generally the vector *HCHAR*) and measures of plan size, age, and ownership (*PCHAR*) were created. As plans are constrained to contract with hospitals in certain geographic areas (defined by SMSA for this analysis), most variables are calculated relative to their direct competitor in the SMSA.

All the variables of *PCHAR* and all but one of the variables of *HCHAR* are discrete. While plan size, plan age, and hospital size are naturally continuous, we create categorical measures to avoid assuming that the effects of these variables are monotonic. Plan size and age are defined by determining if the relevant plan is in the top or bottom 25 percent of the other plans in its SMSA. For the hospital size measure (that is, the number of beds), large hospitals are defined as those in the top quartile of hospitals in the SMSA; small, as in the bottom quartile.

Since the revenues that hospitals earn must, in the long run at least, equal their costs, hospitals must consider their costs in negotiating prices with managed-care plans. This intuition is supported by Melnick et al. (1992), who found that the relative average costs are the strongest predictor of the negotiated price. We will use relative costs as our proxy for price. We will divide total operating costs by the adjusted discharges—taken from the AHA—for each hospital. Then we will calculate the average cost per adjusted discharge (*ACPAD*) for each hospital. Since it is a hospital's *relative* costliness that determines its competitiveness, we will divide each hospital's *ACPAD* by the average *ACPAD* for the SMSA, to create a costliness index.

Plans presumably "learn by doing" in creating their hospital networks, since most of the relevant factors depend mainly on highly local factors. As a result, older plans are likely to have different types of hospital networks from their newer counterparts. Since HMOs tend to be older than PPOs, age categories are likely to have a different effect for each type of plan. Accordingly, we create age categories for each plan type separately; that is, a PPO is "old" if it is in the oldest quartile of PPOs in its SMSA. The vector of hospital characteristics is defined as follows:

prof = 1 if the hospital is for profit, 0 otherwise.

pub = 1 if the hospital is publicly administered, 0 otherwise.

lobeds = 1 if the number of beds is in the bottom quartile, 0 otherwise.

hibeds = 1 if the number of beds is in the top quartile, 0 otherwise.

rcost = expenditures per adjusted discharge divided by the average expenditures per adjusted discharge of hospitals in the SMSA.

hicost =1 if *rcost* is in the top quartile, 0 otherwise.

locost =1 if *rcost* is in the bottom quartile, 0 otherwise.

hsyst = 1 if the hospital is a member in a hospital system, 0 otherwise.

coth = 1 if the hospital is a member of the Council of Teaching Hospitals, 0 otherwise.

te = 1 if the hospital engages in teaching but is not a member of *COTH*, 0 otherwise.

The vector of plan characteristics is defined as follows:

hmo = 1 if the plan is an HMO, 0 otherwise.

pold = 1 if the plan is older than 75 percent of the corresponding type of plans in its SMSA, 0 otherwise.

pnew = 1 if the plan is newer than 75 percent of the plans in its SMSA, 0 otherwise.

pbig = 1 if the plan has more enrollees than 75 percent of the plans in its SMSA, 0 otherwise.

psmall = 1 if the plan has fewer enrollees than 75 percent of the plans in its SMSA, 0 otherwise.

Results

Table 4–1 shows the characteristics of the data collected. There is substantial variability in the number of plans and hospitals in each SMSA, largely reflecting the presence of very large SMSAs, such as Los Angeles, and relatively small ones, such as Sacramento or Tampa, in our data set. The proportion of all hospitals in a network, on average, is much less variable between SMSAs than is the proportion of plans in the SMSA with which each hospital has a contract. The mean probability of a contract tends to lie in the .4–.5 range although there are a few SMSAs in the sample with higher probabilities of approximately .60. Table 4–2 shows that despite the relatively small variability in the mean probability of a contract for most SMSAs, there are large variations at the plan and hospital levels in this probability.

The means and standard deviations of the variable used in the

TABLE 4–1
HOSPITALS, HEALTH CARE PLANS, AND CONTRACTS
IN THIRTEEN SMSAs, 1993

SMSA	Hospitals	Plans	Contracts per Plan	Contracts per Hospital	Contracts per Plan Divided by Number of Hospitals
Boston	54	12	22.0	4.9	.41
Chicago	91	19	38.4	8.0	.42
Dallas	51	9	18.1	3.2	.35
Houston	47	9	14.5	2.8	.31
Los Angeles	191	21	65.2	7.2	.34
Minneapolis	21	7	12.6	4.2	.60
Phoenix	26	14	12.8	6.9	.49
Portland	18	10	7.6	4.2	.42
Sacramento	13	20	7.6	11.6	.58
San Diego	25	23	13.8	12.7	.55
San Francisco	45	21	18.0	8.3	.40
Seattle	15	13	7.6	6.6	.51
Tampa	31	8	9.8	2.5	.32

SOURCE: Author-conducted survey of managed-care plans in 1993.

analysis are provided in table 4–3. The probability of a contract is 0.41; that is, on average plans include roughly 40 percent of the hospitals in the market in their networks. Hospital characteristics such as owner-ship and teaching status are split approximately in expected fashion for urban hospitals, with the majority not for profit and approximately 10 percent of the institutions with intense teaching programs. The high proportion of hospitals that were members of hospital systems reflects both the high proportion of Western SMSAs with the high proportion of for-profit and church-owned hospital systems and the structural changes that have occurred in the markets in the study that have high managed-care penetration.

The coefficients of the three logistic regression models are pre-sented in table 4–4 and the corresponding odds ratios and their 95 percent confidence limits in table 4–5. Since the two sets of results are analytically identical, we will focus our discussions of specific vari-ables on the table 4–4 results.

The omitted SMSA- and plan-level variables improve the fit of the model since there is a statistically significant increase in the log likeli-hood of models with the SMSA and plan dummy variables (table 4–4). A comparison of the estimated coefficients shows that the three regres-

TABLE 4–2
PERCENTAGE OF HOSPITALS IN PLAN NETWORKS AND PERCENTAGE OF
PLANS IN HOSPITAL NETWORKS IN THIRTEEN SMSAs, 1993

SMSA	Percentage of Hospitals in Plan Networks			Percentage of Plans in Hospital Networks		
	Mean	Min.	Max.	Mean	Min.	Max.
Boston	.41	.07	.61	.41	0	.92
Chicago	.42	.14	.73	.42	0	.89
Dallas	.36	.06	.50	.36	0	.77
Houston	.31	.06	.49	.31	0	1
Los Angeles	.38	.04	.54	.38	0	.86
Minneapolis	.60	.24	.86	.60	0	1
Phoenix	.49	.12	.85	.49	0	.79
Portland	.42	.11	.72	.42	.1	.9
Sacramento	.58	.15	.77	.58	.05	.9
San Diego	.55	.04	.88	.55	0	.91
San Francisco	.39	.13	.73	.51	.08	.92
Seattle	.51	.13	.73	.51	.08	.92
Tampa	.31	.13	.52	.31	0	.75

SOURCE: Author-conducted survey of managed-care plans in 1993.

sion models yield similar results, so that the variables in the model must be statistically independent of the SMSA and plan variables that are proxied by the dummy variables in the respective models. In addition, the results are seen to be reassuringly robust, in that the *FE* does not decrease the significance of the variables in the model. Model 1 (uncorrelated residuals) and model 2 (SMSA fixed effects) are generally similar in the patterns they reveal regarding the plan characteristics that affect the probability of a contract. A summary of the key results follows:

• Managed-care plans have a clear preference for not-for-profit hospitals. Surprisingly, they even prefer public hospitals to for-profit ones.

• Size is important. Larger hospitals have a higher probability of contracting than medium-sized hospitals, and they, in turn, are preferred over small hospitals.

• Teaching hospitals are less likely to belong to hospital networks; hospitals with the most intense teaching programs, members of the Council of Teaching Hospitals, are the least likely to contract with managed-care plans.

• Membership in a hospital system does not affect the probability of a contract.

TABLE 4–3

CHARACTERISTICS OF HOSPITALS AND HEALTH CARE PLANS FOR
THIRTEEN SMSAs, 1993

Variable	Mean	Standard Deviation
Contract	.41	.49
For-profit	.29	.46
Public	.12	.34
Smallest-quartile hospital	.26	.44
Largest-quartile hospital	.23	.42
Relative cost index	.95	.48
System vs. nonsystem	.57	.52
Member of Council of Teaching Hospitals	.09	.29
Other teaching hospitals	.18	.38
HMO	.48	.48
Oldest-quartile plan in SMSA	.15	.36
Newest-quartile plan in SMSA	.44	.53
Smallest-quartile plan in SMSA	.27	.45
Largest-quartile plan in SMSA	.33	.47

SOURCE: Author-conducted survey of managed-care plans 1993.

• Hospitals that have higher relative costs consistently have a lower probability of contracting, but insignificantly so.

• HMOs have smaller networks than PPOs.

• The oldest plans in each SMSA have far fewer contracts than do plans that have a shorter history in an SMSA, controlling for plan enrollment.

• The smallest plans, those in the lowest quartile, tend to have fewer contracts.

We regressed the relative cost index against all the other hospital characteristics to test whether the observed insignificant relationship between relative costs and the probability of a contract was due to multicollinearity. We then used the residual from this equation in the logistic regression. The results were substantially unchanged (data not shown).

As a further investigation into the unexpected effect of relative costs on contracting, we investigated whether there may be a nonmonotonic relationship between costs and the probability of a contract. Tables 4–6 and 4–7 show the regression results corresponding to model 1 (no error structure) and the corresponding odds ratios. The results with SMSA and plan fixed-effect models were essentially the same (data not shown). The results show that both the highest- and the low-

TABLE 4–4

LOGISTIC REGRESSION MODELS OF HOSPITALS AND HEALTH CARE PLANS
FOR THIRTEEN SMSAs, 1993

Variable	No Error Structure[a]	SMSA Fixed Effects[a]	Plan Fixed Effects[a]
For-profit	−.98	−.93	−1.02
Public	−.66	−.77	−.83
Smallest-quartile hospital	−.51	−.55	−.06
Largest-quartile hospital	.62	.61	.70
Relative cost index	−.004*	−.01*	−.01*
System	−.013*	−.09*	.07*
Member of Council of Teaching Hospitals	−.58	−.52	−.61
Other teaching hospitals	−.53	−.51	−.60
HMO vs. non-HMO	−.22	−.19	NA
Oldest-quartile plan in SMSA	−.25	−.25	NA
Newest-quartile plan in SMSA	.04	.02*	NA
Smallest-quartile plan in SMSA	−.21	−.19	NA
Largest-quartile plan in SMSA	−.10	−.02*	NA
Constant	.32	.03	.66

NA = not applicable.
* = not statistically significant at the 0.05 level. All other coefficients are significant.
a. Coefficient (z).
SOURCE: Author-conducted survey of managed-care plans, 1993.

est-cost hospitals are significantly less likely to get contracts. All else being equal, a hospital in the lowest-cost quartile within an SMSA would be 30 percent less likely to get a contract than the group with average costs (in the middle 50 percent). The effect of being in the highest-cost quartile is less dramatic, approximately reducing the probability of a contract by 20 percent.

Discussion and Implications

As the results show, managed-care contracting with hospitals follows systematic patterns. Clearly, important SMSA- and plan-level variables have been omitted from our analysis, not surprisingly given the limited set of variables included in this analysis. We will discuss below the

TABLE 4–5

ODDS RATIO IN LOGISTIC REGRESSION MODELS OF HOSPITALS AND
HEALTH CARE PLANS FOR THIRTEEN SMSAS, 1993

Variable	Model 1		Model 2		Model 3	
	Odds ratio	95% confidence	Odds ratio	95% confidence	Odds ratio	95% confidence
For-profit vs. not-for-profit	.38	.34–.42	.39	.35–.44	.36	.32–.41
Public vs. not-for-profit	.52	.48–.59	.46	.4–.54	.44	.37–.51
Smallest-quartile hospital vs. interquartile hospitals	.63	.54–.67	.58	.51–.64	.55	.49–.61
Largest-quartile hospital vs. interquartile hospitals	1.86	1.66–2.06	1.84	1.63–2.16	2.04	1.81–2.26
Relative cost index	.99	.91–1.09	.99	.91–1.08	.99	.89–1.08
System vs. nonsystem	1.01	.91–1.12	.92	.84–1.0	.93	.85–1.0
Member of Council of Teaching Hospitals vs. nonteaching	.56	.47–.67	.59	.49–.71	.54	.45–.66
Other teaching hospitals vs. nonteaching	.59	.52–.66	.60	.53–.68	.55	.49–.63
HMO vs. non-HMO	.81	.74–.87	.82	.76–.90	NA	NA
Oldest-quartile in SMSA vs. interquartile plan	.78	.69–.87	.78	.69–.87	NA	NA
Newest-quartile in SMSA vs. interquartile plan	1.04	.92–1.16	1.03	.89–1.17	NA	NA
Smallest-quartile in SMSA vs. interquartile plan	.81	.72–.91	.93	.88–1.07	NA	NA
Largest-quartile in SMSA vs. interquartile plan	.91	.82–1.00	.98	.88–1.08	NA	NA

NA = not applicable.
SOURCE: Author-conducted survey of managed-care plans, 1993.

types of additional variables that we intend to add in the analysis stage
of these data.

Some of the results are consistent with our initial expectations,
and others are clearly surprises. One surprise is the extent to which
managed-care plans prefer not to contract with for-profit hospitals. A
for-profit hospital, all else being equal, has less than 40 percent the
probability of having a contract that a not-for-profit hospital has. So
strong is this effect that public hospitals, usually regarded as the hospitals of last resort, are more likely to get managed-care contracts than

TABLE 4–6

"SPLIT COST" REGRESSION OF HOSPITALS AND HEALTH CARE PLANS FOR
THIRTEEN SMSAs, 1993

Plan	Coefficient
For-profit	− .98
Public	− .67
Smallest-quartile hospital	− .47
Largest-quartile hospital	.60
Low cost	− .36
High cost	− .24
System	.01*
Member of Council of Teaching Hospitals	− .50
Other teaching hospitals	− .51
HMO vs. non-HMO	− .22
Oldest-quartile plan in SMSA	− .24
Newest-quartile plan in SMSA	.06*
Smallest-quartile plan in SMSA	− .22
Largest-quartile plan in SMSA	− .11
Constant	.44

* = not statistically significant at the 0.05 level. All other coefficients are significant.
SOURCE: Author-conducted survey of managed-care plans, 1993.

for-profit ones are. One may hypothesize several alternative explanations for this phenomenon. One is that for-profits are less willing to agree to concessions, either in the area of price or in other areas, than not-for-profits are. This explanation may be plausible, since for-profits are presumably profit maximizers and many models of the utility function of not-for-profit hospitals includes volume. This explanation also implies that not-for-profit hospitals may be willing to agree to price concessions to maintain volume that for-profits would not. Another possibility is that the medical staffs of for-profit hospitals are narrower and, therefore, do not fit in as well into the physician networks the managed-care plans are creating. A third alternative is that the plan choice reflects consumer demand, which prefers not-for-profit hospitals, perhaps reflecting an assessment of the quality of care at these institutions. Yet another possibility is that these results reflect the preferences of not-for-profit managed-care plans, which, in turn, employers appear to prefer (Wholey, Feldman, and Christianson 1995). Clearly, we should try to determine the degree to which these alternatives explain the observed preference of not-for-profit hospitals over their for-profit competitors.

The observed preference for larger hospitals is expected. Substan-

TABLE 4–7
Odds Ratio from "Split Cost" Regression of Hospitals and
Health Care Plans for Thirteen SMSAs, 1993

Plan	Odds Ratio	95% Confidence Interval
For-profit vs. not-for-profit	.38	.34–.42
Public vs. not-for-profit	.51	.44–.59
Smallest-quartile hospital vs. interquartile hospitals	.63	.56–.70
Largest-quartile hospital vs. interquartile hospitals	1.82	1.62–2.06
Low cost vs. medium cost	.70	.63–.79
High cost vs. medium cost	.78	.70–.88
System vs. nonsystem	1.01	.92–1.10
Member of Council of Teaching Hospitals vs. nonteaching	.61	.51–.73
Other teaching hospitals vs. nonteaching	.60	.53–.67
HMO vs. non-HMO	.80	.74–.87
Oldest-quartile in SMSA vs. interquartile plan	.78	.70–.88
Newest-quartile in SMSA vs. interquartile plan	1.06	.93–1.21
Smallest-quartile in SMSA vs. interquartile plan	.80	.72–.90
Largest-quartile in SMSA vs. interquartile plan	.89	.81–.99

Source: Author-conducted survey of managed-care plans, 1993.

tial anecdotal evidence suggests that managed-care plans preferred the service breadth (and possibly the reputation for higher quality) available at larger hospitals. The observed tendency to add new services in response to the competitive pressures of managed care (Zwanziger, Melnick, and Simonson 1996) appears to be a response to this preference. This tendency obviously places small urban hospitals at a disadvantage, and it would be important to confirm that size is a proxy for service breadth.

Teaching hospitals are substantially less likely to have contracts than are the corresponding nonteaching hospitals (somewhat more than 50 percent of the probability). This effect is independent of the relative costliness. A possible explanation for that effect is that variables highly correlated with teaching status (which plans tend to disfavor) are omitted. Teaching hospitals, for example, may have payer mixes (high proportion of Medicaid or uninsured patients), or inner-city locations that plan enrollees do not like. Alternatively, these hospitals may tend to have higher prices than their nonteaching counterparts, or their medical staffs may be difficult to integrate into plans' physician networks. Finally, there may, on net, be a perception of lower quality of care in teaching hospitals because of the involvement of residents and interns in patient care.

The plan effects are all plausible. HMOs with their greater restrictiveness would be expected to have smaller hospital networks. Plans tend to prune their networks over time (by approximately 20 percent). Small plans tend to have smaller networks, possibly reflecting the fact that they may serve only a portion of the metropolitan area.

We have deferred discussion of the two most intriguing findings: the fact that neither system membership nor relative costs have a significant effect on the probability of a contract. One might expect that the additional market power created by system membership would translate into a higher probability of a contract. If anything, the opposite is true, with system hospitals somewhat less likely to have contracts. This finding suggests either that systems do not have market power or that they use it for purposes other than increasing their contracting, such as increasing the prices they receive. Alternatively, system hospitals may have joined a system because they were in a weak position (since the model controls for many hospital characteristics, these would have to be factors that are both omitted and result in a weak market position such as a reputation for poor quality). Finally, our system variable may be inappropriately defined, with local systems—that is, systems concentrated in a given area—behaving differently from national or regional systems that do not have enough concentration in any given area to exert substantial market power.

The most unexpected result was the insignificance of the relative cost index. This result is consistent with the Feldman et al. (1990) study, which showed that plans' contracting decision was independent of average costs, but that they focused their efforts on channeling their beneficiaries to lower-cost hospitals in their network. Measurement error hampered the analysis. The variable of importance is the offering price, not relative cost, but a previous study (Melnick et al. 1992) suggested that mean costs could serve as a partial proxy for prices. The results implied that while higher costs act as a deterrent to getting a contract, that relationship is not monotonic, with the lowest-cost hospitals also less likely to get contracts. Since offering price is almost certainly a critical factor in securing a contract, the fact that the cost index does not behave as expected means that in general the two are poorly correlated. There must then be other systematic or random factors that obscure the relationship between average costs and offering price. A measurement error will always occur since we are using available variables as proxies for prices. We may be able to reduce this error by including other factors that mediate the relationship between average cost and price. These include case mixture; the financial pressure of Medicare, Medicaid, and uncompensated care; and the competitiveness of both the hospital and the plan markets. The fact that low costs act as a deterrent to contracting may suggest either that plans use costs as quality proxies or that low costs are correlated with other factors that the public does not like. Elucidating these relationships is a critical area of development for this study.

This study, a preliminary analysis using a new type of data set, studies the factors affecting managed-care contracting. Some patterns are clearly evident even now. They provide a useful means of generating new hypotheses to deepen our understanding of the functioning of these markets. Studies expanding on the current one should attempt to incorporate important variables that were excluded, for example, T measures of quality and a more sensitive measure of system membership that quantifies the degree to which the system possesses market power. In addition, critical issues concerning the "architecture" of hospital networks remain, such as the degree of system coordination and the weight that managed-care plans place on geographic separation when designing their hospital networks. An understanding of these dynamics would provide an empirical underpinning to antitrust policy. Much important work remains to be done.

References

Brown, E. R., M. R. Cousineau, and W. T. Price. 1985. "Competing for Med-Cal Business: Why Hospitals Did and Did Not, Get Contracts." *Inquiry* 22: 237–50.

Chernew, M. 1993. "The Impact of Managed Care on the Structure of the Market for Hospital Services." Mimeo, University of Michigan.

Eckholm, E. 1994. "While Congress Remains Silent, Health Care Transforms Itself." *New York Times*, December 18.

Farley, D. E. 1985. "Competition among Hospitals: Market Structure and Its Relation to Utilization, Costs, and Financial Position." Research Note 7, Hospital Studies Program, National Center for Health Services Research and Health Care Technology Assessment.

Feldman, R., H. C. Chan, J. Kralewski, B. Dowd, and J. Shapiro. 1990. "Effect of HMOs on the Creation of Competitive Markets for Hospital Services." *Journal of Health Economics* 9: 207–22.

Feldman, R., and B. Dowd. 1986. "Is There a Competitive Market for Hospital Services?" *Journal of Health Economics* 5(3): 277–92.

Gruber, J. 1994. "The Effect of Competitive Pressure on Charity: Hospital Responses to Price Shopping in California." *Journal of Health Economics* 13: 183–212.

Jensen, G. A., M. A. Morrisey, S. Gaffney, and D. K. Liston. 1997. "The New Dominance of Managed Care: Insurance Trends in the 1990s." *Health Affairs* (Winter): 125–36.

Johns, L. 1989. "Selective Contracting in California: An Update." *Inquiry* 26: 345–53.

Johns, L., R. A. Derzon, and M. D. Anderson. 1985. "Selective Contracting in California: Early Effects and Policy Implications." *Inquiry* 22: 24–32.

Joskow, P. L. 1980. "The Effects of Competition and Regulation on Hospital Bed Supply and the Reservation Quality of the Hospital." *Bell Journal of Economics* 11: 195–221.

Luft, H., J. Robinson, D. Garnick, S. Maerki, and S. McPhee. 1986. "The Role of Specialized Clinical Services in Competition among Hospitals." *Inquiry* 23: 83–94.

Luft, J. S., and S. C. Maerki. 1984–1985. "Competitive Potential of Hospitals and Their Neighbors." *Contemporary Policy Issues* 3: 89–102.

McLaughlin, C. G. 1988. "Market Responses to HMOs: Price Competition or Rivalry?" *Inquiry* 25: 207–18.

Melnick, G. A., and J. Zwanziger. 1988. "Hospital Behavior under Competition and Cost Containment Policies: The California Experience, 1980 to 1985." *Journal of the American Medical Association* 260: 2669–75.

Melnick, G., J. Zwanziger, A. Bamezai, and R. Pattison. 1992. "The Effects of Market Structure and Bargaining Position on Hospital Prices." *Journal of Health Economics* 11 (3): 217–33.

Melnick, G. A., J. Zwanziger, and A. Verity-Guerra. 1989. "The Growth and Effects of Hospital Selective Contracting." *Health Care Management Review* 14 (3): 57–64.

Mennemeyer, S. T., and L. Olinger. 1989. "Selective Contracting in California: Its Effects on Hospital Finances." *Inquiry* 26 (4): 442–47.

Robinson, J. C. 1991. "HMO Market Penetration and Hospital Cost Inflation in California." *Journal of the American Medical Association* 266 (19): 2719–23.

Robinson, J., and H. Luft. 1985. "Competition and the Cost of Hospital Care, 1972 to 1982." *Journal of the American Medical Association* 257 (23): 3241–45.

Securities Data Company. 1994. Newark, N.J.

Simon, C. J., and P. H. Born. 1996. "Physician Earning in a Changing Managed Care Environment." *Health Affairs* 15 (Fall): 124–33.

Wholey, D., R. Feldman, and J. B. Christianson. 1995. "The Effect of Market Structure on HMO Premiums." *Journal of Health Economics* 14: 81–105.

Wilson, G. W., and J. M. Jadlow. 1982. "Competition, Profit Incentives and Technical Efficiency in the Provision of Nuclear Medicine Services." *Bell Journal of Economics* 13 (Autumn).

Zwanziger, J., and G. Melnick. 1988. "The Effects of Hospital Competition and the Medicare PPS Program on Hospital Cost Behavior in California." *Journal of Health Economics* 7 (4): 301–20.

Zwanziger, J., G. A. Melnick, and L. Simonson. 1996. "Differentiation and Specialization in the California Hospital Industry 1983–1988." *Medical Care* 34: 361–72.

5
Managed Care and the Physician Marketplace

Carol J. Simon, William D. White, Patricia Born, and David Dranove

The growth of managed care has dominated recent changes in the medical marketplace. As of 1995, more than 120 million Americans were enrolled in a health maintenance organization (HMO) or preferred provider organization (PPO), up from 10 million in 1982 (AMCRA 1995). By 1995, more than 83 percent of patient-care physicians had at least one managed-care contract (Emmons and Simon 1996). There is a growing body of evidence that suggests that managed care is changing the market for physician services and, in particular, is altering the relative emphasis on specialty and primary care (Anders 1995; Morgan 1994; Page 1994; and Rosenthal 1995). This has far-reaching implications for the operation of the health care system and work force policy. In this chapter, we use nationally representative data on physicians to evaluate economic evidence of changes in the supply of and demand for primary care and specialist physicians over the past decade. We build on Simon and Born's 1996 work on physician compensation: first, by extending the analysis to a multivariate framework, and second, by examining adjustments in physician supply that we would expect to follow changes in compensation.

We make use of the fact that, while virtually all regions in the United States have witnessed the growth of managed care, the rate of growth and the levels of managed-care penetration in the marketplace are quite geographically varied. First, we examine the relationship be-

This research was undertaken while Patricia Born was a senior economist at the American Medical Association, Center for Health Policy Research. This chapter reflects the opinions of the authors and should not be interpreted as representing the policies or positions of the American Medical Association, the University of Illinois, Northwestern University, or the Agency for Health Care Policy and Research.

tween state-level managed-care penetration and the corresponding rate of growth in the incomes of primary care and specialty physicians. Our analysis of physician income spans the period between 1985 and 1994. Second, we examine the relationship between managed-care penetration and changes in the numbers of primary care and specialty physicians per capita for the same period. Finally, we consider national trends in the matches of graduating U.S. medical school seniors with specialty programs for the period 1989–1997.

We find that major adjustments are underway in the markets for primary care physicians and specialists, and that market forces associated with the growth of managed care may be an important contributing factor. We close with a discussion of the latest evidence on trends in the physician marketplace and consider the public policy implications of our findings.

Background

A major feature of U.S. medicine has been the high reliance on medical specialists to deliver patient care. Currently, specialists account for about 70 percent of all active physicians in the United States (Marder et al. 1988; Kindig et al. 1993). It is frequently asserted that reliance on specialists may increase the costs of care because they are more expensive to train than are primary care physicians and because they may employ more expensive treatment styles. In addition, extensive use of specialists may lead to fragmentation of care and may reduce continuity and access (Eisenberg 1994; Grumbach and Lee 1991; Moore 1994; Reinhardt 1994; Schroeder 1994; and Wennberg et al. 1993).

There are several reasons why managed care might economize on the use of physician services and alter the compensation of both primary care physicians and specialists. Under managed care the locus of decision making about where care is received and what care is obtained is shifted from individual patients and their physicians toward insurers and employers. Under traditional fee-for-service indemnity policies, most patients have been insulated from the true price of care because of the prevalence of comprehensive benefits and low copayments and deductibles. In contrast, managed-care plans realize the full amount of any cost savings. Accordingly, they have strong incentives to be cost-conscious shoppers for care. Managed-care plans may also be better able to realize economies of scale in gathering information about price and using large databases to evaluate the efficacy of using alternative treatments and types of personnel. Altogether, this suggests that managed-care plans should be more price sensitive and generally less willing to pay for more expensive, or less effective, medical services.

Managed-care plans have sought directly to control use of specialists through utilization review and reliance on primary care physicians as "gatekeepers" (Franks et al. 1992). Plans can also seek out providers with relatively low-cost treatment styles. To the extent that these treatment styles are associated with greater use of primary and preventive care, this behavior may affect relative demand for primary care versus specialist physicians. We expect these factors simultaneously to boost the compensation and employment of primary care physicians while reducing the compensation and employment of specialists.

There is limited evidence about the effect of managed care on physician demand. A number of studies have shown that staff model HMOs use fewer specialists per capita than do other patient care settings (Arnould et al. 1984; Dial et al. 1995; Manning et al. 1984; and Gamliel et al. 1995). Care must be exercised, however, in extrapolating findings for staff HMOs to the broader marketplace (Hart et al. 1997). In particular, staff model HMOs make up a small fraction of the managed-care market. Other forms of managed care—including IPAs, PPOs, and point-of-service plans—have been growing much more rapidly. Work force requirements under other forms of managed care are not well documented (Kronick et al. 1993), and recent studies suggest they may not significantly alter demand for physician services (Congressional Budget Office 1994; Goldman 1995).

The results of the staffing studies are also confounded by patient sorting. There is substantial evidence that relatively healthier individuals choose to enroll in managed care (Hellinger 1995; Luft 1991). As such, these patients would have used fewer health care services in any setting. If the primary effect of managed care is simply to sort patients based on their health status, the total demand for various types of physician services at the market level may be unaffected, even though physician work force requirements might vary substantially across different types of managed-care plans.

Economic Implications for Physicians. In the short run, changes in the demand for physician services will be reflected most rapidly in the form of changes in physician earnings. An increase in the demand for primary care services would give rise to a scarcity of primary care physicians. Primary care earnings would rise not only because existing primary care physicians would be delivering more services, but because competing managed-care plans and other payers would tend to bid up fees and remuneration.

Similarly, a decline in the demand for specialty care would generate a surfeit of specialists. Specialist compensation would be depressed as patient volumes fell and specialists were forced to reduce fees to obtain contracts with payers or employers. If specialists can induce demand for their services, then the effect of declining prices may be partially offset by prescribing higher levels of services. Recent evidence, however, suggests that specialists could not induce enough demand to make up more than a small portion of the lost income (Gaynor 1994; McGuire and Pauly 1991).

Taken together, we would expect that in those markets with high managed-care penetration, the incomes of specialists would fall relative to the incomes of primary care physicians. Such a finding would be consistent with an increase in demand for primary care physicians, a reduction in demand for specialists, or both.

Short-run changes in income will generate incentives for physicians to make longer run adjustments in their practices. Physicians who are in markets where demand is shrinking may look to relocate to markets where incomes are stable or growing. We would also expect an increase in the number of newly trained physicians electing to enter primary care, as well as a possible rise in the number of practicing specialists switching to primary care. Studies have found that physician choices of specialty training may be quite sensitive to expected lifetime earnings, suggesting that these long-run adjustments could be quite profound (McKay 1990; Rosenthal et al. 1994).

Methods Overview. We draw on three types of evidence to gauge the effect of managed care on the physician marketplace. First, we examine the relationship between changes in managed-care penetration and rate of growth of primary care and specialty physicians' incomes. Such an analysis may be conducted across plans—that is, comparing incomes of physicians in and out of managed-care plans—or across geographic areas—that is, comparing incomes of physicians across areas with different levels of managed-care penetration. Plan-level analysis cannot readily distinguish between differences that derive from managed care and those that arise because physicians and patients sort themselves into managed-care organizations according to other, uncontrolled attributes. Thus, we prefer to look across geographic areas.

We analyze physician incomes and location at the state level for the period 1985 to 1994. States are sufficiently diverse in their populations' sociodemographic characteristics, their physicians' characteristics, and their levels of managed-care penetration to support a meaningful analysis. The study period affords us the ability to examine the physician marketplace during a period of rapid and widespread managed-care growth, while utilizing recently available information on physician earnings. States are also large enough to minimize biases that may result from patient border crossing. One limitation of state data is that managed-care growth has been concentrated in larger urban areas, and some states have a mix of rural and urban populations. As a result, intrastate adjustments in physician location may occur that will not be identified in our analysis of supply trends. To the extent that intrastate variation in managed-care penetration is masked by a state-level analysis, our findings may understate the true effect of managed care.

We begin by examining the relationship between changes in managed-care penetration and the compensation of physicians. Physicians have historically enjoyed strong earnings growth. Beginning in the 1990s, however, growth rates slowed and became more variable. In 1994, there was a broad-based decline in physician earnings. We document changes in the level and distribution of earnings for primary care physicians (PCPs) and specialists with an eye toward examining the influence of major trends in managed care . We then turn to a statistical analysis of the effect of managed-care growth on annualized rates of growth in incomes of primary care and specialty physicians. We compute regression-adjusted income changes to control explicitly for the effect of changes in state-specific socioeconomic variables—that is, population demographics, insurance status, and other factors that affect demand for physician services—over the study period. We analyze changes in income, rather than income levels, in order to minimize the effect of uncontrolled or unobserved state-level factors that are unrelated to managed-care growth but that may confound a cross-sectional analysis.

Second, we explore supply responses. We examine the relationship between changes in managed-care penetration and annualized rates of growth of the number of primary care and specialty physicians per capita. Again, we conduct this analysis at the state level for the period 1985–1994 and use multivariate regression to control for factors unrelated to the growth of managed care. We expect to find changes in the primary care physician-to-population ratio positively related to the spread of managed care, and growth in specialist physician-to-population ratios negatively related to managed care. Physicians incur substantial costs in relocating or changing established practices; hence we expect that adjustments in the numbers of physicians will occur less rapidly than adjustments in compensation.

Finally, we examine trends in choices of specialty training by U.S. medical school seniors using data from the National Residency Matching Program for the period 1985–1996. To the extent recent regional changes portend long-term national trends, we expect to find medical students increasingly selecting residencies in primary care. Our analysis of specialty choices of new medical graduates is limited to national data.

Data

We use data from the American Medical Association's (AMA) Socio-economic Monitoring System (SMS) surveys to measure physicians' incomes and involvement in managed care.

Physician Income. The SMS is an annual telephone survey of nonfederal, post-residency physicians, active for twenty hours or more a week in patient care. The SMS is designed to be representative of the patient-care physician population. It has a 60–70 percent response rate, and it gathers approximately 4,000 responses annually, corresponding to 1 percent of patient-care physicians. Responses are weighted for nonresponse bias by comparing SMS sample frequencies to the distributions of physicians in the AMA Masterfile according to specialty, years of experience, AMA membership, and board certification status. The AMA Masterfile includes data on specialty, location, and practice status of all known physicians in the United States.

Income is defined as net practice income after expenses and before taxes, including contributions into deferred compensation plans, but excluding investment income. Income numbers are converted to 1994 inflation-adjusted levels, using the consumer price index.

Specialty Classification. Specialty categories can be broad (for example, internal medicine) or narrow (for example, pediatric nephrology). We define three categories for our analyses of incomes and location. Categories are defined to capture maximum variation in the effect of managed care on different "types" of physicians, while generating sufficient sample sizes to support a state-level analysis. We classify physicians as either: (1) primary care physicians (PCPs), defined as physicians practicing in general or family practice, general internal medicine, and pediatrics; (2) subspecialists, defined as physicians practicing in either a surgical or medical specialty (such as orthopaedic surgeons and cardiologists), and who typically provide small amounts of primary care; or (3) RAPs—radiologists, anesthesiologists, and pathologists. We distinguish RAPs from other specialists because they provide virtually no primary care, their services are generally demanded only upon referral, and they may be replaced with relatively less disruption to continuity of care. As a result, RAPs may be most vulnerable to cost-cutting efforts by managed-care organizations. RAP physicians are also historically closely associated with inpatient hospital services. Research has shown that one of the most significant effects of managed care is to reduce utilization of inpatient hospital services (Congressional Budget Office 1994).

Our three specialty classifications encompass 81 percent of all patient care physicians. Physicians with specialties in obstetrics and gynecology, emergency medicine, and psychiatry are excluded from the analysis for two reasons. First, it is more difficult to predict the effect of managed care on these groups. For example, OB-GYNs and emergency medicine physicians frequently deliver a mixture of primary and specialty care. The net effect of managed care on these practices is ambiguous. Second, none of these specialties constitutes more than 6 percent of the SMS physician population, yielding too few physicians at the state level to support separate analysis of the specialty. Aggregating these specialties would produce groups that had too much intragroup heterogeneity.

We obtain each physician's self-designated specialty—namely, the specialty from which the physician derives most of his or her practice income—from the SMS survey. In 1994, 33 percent of all physicians were in primary care, 29 percent were specialists, and 19 percent were RAPs. For the fifty states and the District of Columbia, our three-way classification of physicians yields a potential total of 153 observations. In the multivariate regressions, state-specialty categories with fewer than five observations are dropped from the analysis, leaving us with a total of 140 usable observations.

Measuring Managed-Care Penetration. We use the SMS to construct measures of state-level managed-care penetration. One major advantage of SMS survey data is that they capture information on a wide range of different types of managed-care delivery systems—in particular, newer hybrid network forms that rely on selective contracting. The SMS identifies (1) employment in staff-model HMOs, (2) contracting with various types of managed-care plans (MCOs), and (3) the share of physician practice revenues coming from these contracts. Previous research has been forced to focus exclusively on the HMO enrollment by state, owing to the lack of reliable data on the market shares of other forms of managed care. HMOs, however, make up less than half the MCO market.

From the SMS, we estimate the percentage of physician revenue in each state that is derived from all MCO contracts and define this to be our indicator of the economic importance of managed care. Our definition excludes traditional indemnity plans that rely only on forms of utilization and preauthorization review to "manage" care.

101

FIGURE 5–1
DISTRIBUTION OF VALUES OF STATE-LEVEL MANAGED-CARE
PENETRATION, 1985 AND 1994

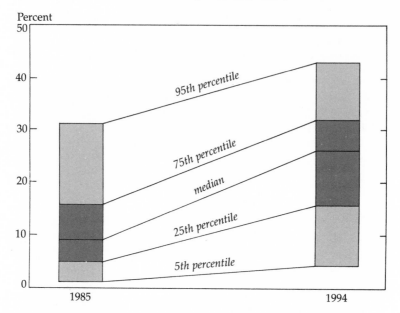

SOURCE: Authors.

As noted above, there is considerable geographic variation in the level of managed-care penetration across states and in the growth that has occurred in the past decade. Figure 5–1 illustrates the distribution of values of state-level managed-care penetration, in 1985 and 1994.

Physician Earnings and Managed Care

The effect of managed care on physician compensation is best understood against a backdrop of historic trends in physician compensation.

Trends in the Level and Distribution of Physician Earnings. Figure 5–2 illustrates the growth in average physician income over the past decade, while figures 5–3 through 5–5 illustrate trends in the average level of compensation and intraspecialty variation in earnings for each of our specialty groups.

Between 1985 and 1994 average real (inflation-adjusted) physician income rose cumulatively by 26 percent. This implies that physician

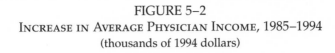

FIGURE 5–2
INCREASE IN AVERAGE PHYSICIAN INCOME, 1985–1994
(thousands of 1994 dollars)

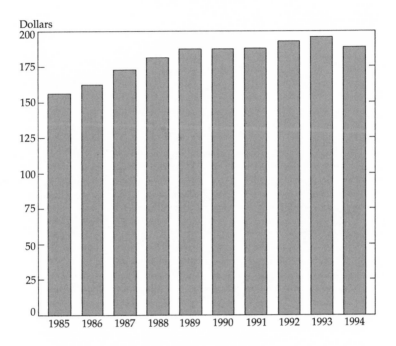

SOURCE: Authors' calculations based on AMA SMS data.

earnings rose at an annual rate that was 2 percent higher than the average rate of inflation. It is noteworthy that during this same period, trends in real wages for the U.S. work force were essentially flat. There is a distinct change in the trends between the 1980s and 1990s. Prior to 1990, physician earnings rose steadily at an average annual rate of 3.1 percent, while after 1990 the annual increases averaged less than 1 percent and year-to-year changes were more volatile. Between 1993 and 1994, average earnings fell by 3.8 percent—marking the first decline in more than a decade.

Across all years, primary care physicians reported the lowest level of earnings and also averaged the lowest growth in earnings, rising 19 percent from 1985–1993 before falling by 2 percent in 1994. Specialists enjoyed a 29 percent increase in real compensation between 1985 and 1993, and they suffered a 7 percent decline in 1994. Hospital-based

FIGURE 5–3

INCOME DISTRIBUTION OF PRIMARY CARE PHYSICIANS, 1985–1994

(thousands of 1994 dollars)

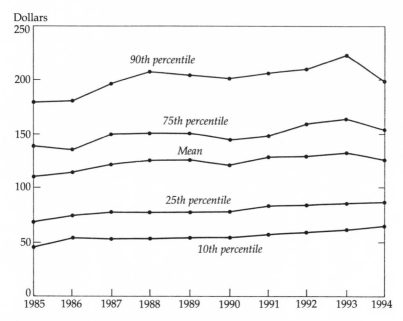

SOURCE: Authors' calculations based on AMA SMS data, 1985–1994.

RAPs saw average earnings climb 25 percent from 1985–1993 and fall 6 percent in 1994.

Managed care may be expected to narrow earnings differentials between primary care physicians and specialists. Indeed, specialist earnings began the study period at 167 percent of primary care earnings, peaked in 1990 at 189 percent of PCP income, and fell to 173 percent of PCP earnings in 1994.

Utilization review, discounts off fees, and payment schemes that reward physicians for parsimonious use of services might be expected disproportionately to affect physicians at the upper end of the earnings distribution—that is, those who perform more services, more expensive services, and more highly remunerated services. This is borne out in our data. PCPs and specialists who were in the lowest stratum of the earnings distributions had steady earnings growth through 1993. Growth continued for lower-paid PCPs in 1994, but incomes declined among the lower-paid specialists. The income distribution generally widened for all specialty groups in the late 1980s and narrowed in the

104

FIGURE 5–4
INCOME DISTRIBUTION OF SPECIALISTS, 1985–1994
(thousands of 1994 dollars)

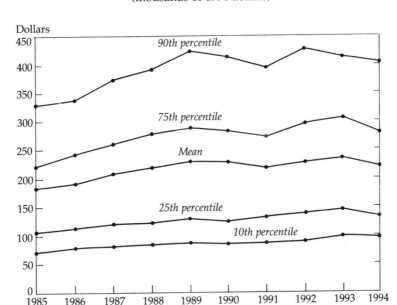

SOURCE: Authors' calculations based on AMA SMS data.

1990s. Specialists and RAPs who were in the upper earnings stratum led the decline in earnings. Earnings began to fall for the most highly compensated RAPs as early as 1991, while the earnings of highly paid specialists had stagnated by 1990 and fallen from 1992–1994. This is noteworthy since Medicare's resource-based relative value system, which was implemented in 1992, aimed at reducing compensation for procedures and increasing remuneration for primary care visits.

Is Managed Care behind the Earnings Trends? We begin by examining the relationship between changes in managed-care penetration and annualized rates of growth in the earnings of primary care and specialty physicians using multivariate regression. Because of the sharp change in earnings trends in 1994, we construct our analysis so that we can identify whether the factors that affected physician income differed in 1994 from what they were in previous years. Specifically, we analyze the influence of managed-care penetration on physician earn-

105

FIGURE 5–5
INCOME DISTRIBUTION OF RAPs, 1985–1994
(thousands of 1994 dollars)

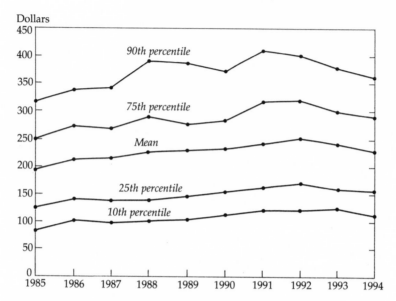

SOURCE: Authors' calculations based on AMA SMS data.

ings growth over 1985–1993 and separately for the period 1993–1994.[1]

We measure the effect of managed care first by ranking states on the basis of average managed-care penetration between 1985 and 1993 and constructing indicator variables that correspond to each quartile. For example, states such as Arkansas and Wyoming, where there has been little managed care, score a value of 1 for the indicator variable corresponding to the lowest managed-care quartile, and zeros in the other three quartile indicators. Our results are robust with respect to alternative transformations of the managed-care variables. Table 5–1 reports the states and managed-care penetration rates associated with each quartile.

Explanatory variables include indicators of state-level managed-care penetration and controls for other factors affecting the demand for physician services. Control variables are designed to capture the

1. We experimented with other subperiod analyses, as well. There were small but not uniformly statistically significant differences in the relation between income and managed care, using 1985–1990 and 1991–1993 as distinct subperiods.

TABLE 5–1
MANAGED-CARE PENETRATION BY QUARTILE, 1985–1994
(percent)

Managed-Care Quartile	Average Managed-Care Penetration
First quartile: Arkansas, Kentucky, Idaho, Maine, Mississippi, Montana, New Hampshire, North Carolina, North Dakota, South Carolina, South Dakota, West Virginia, Vermont	1.1–9.8
Second quartile: D.C., Georgia, Illinois, Indiana, Iowa, Louisiana, Nebraska, New Jersey, New York, Pennsylvania, Texas, Virginia	10.7–17.0
Third quartile: Alabama, Connecticut, Delaware, Florida, Hawaii, Kansas, Maryland, Michigan, Missouri, Ohio, Oklahoma, Tennessee	18.2–20.8
Fourth quartile: Arizona, California, Colorado, Massachusetts, Minnesota, New Mexico, Nevada, Oregon, Rhode Island, Utah, Washington, Wisconsin	22.5–38.7

SOURCE: Authors' calculations based on SMS 1985–1994 surveys.

effects of population age, income, and insurance status on physician earnings. Controls include the percentage of the population under the age of five, the percentage of the population over the age of sixty-five, the percentage that is nonwhite, the percentage that is urban, percentage uninsured, and per capita income.

We compute and report regression-adjusted income changes by managed-care quartile. Estimated coefficients on the indicator variables in the multivariate regressions reflect the differential effect of managed care on physician incomes across quartiles.

We estimate separate regression equations for each of the three specialty groups. Our dependent variable is the change in median physician income, by state and specialty group. We use median income, in lieu of mean income, to attenuate the influence of outliers. We recognize that if managed care has had a greater influence on physicians in the upper income deciles, using the median will underestimate the actual effects of managed care. There is some evidence in the descriptive analysis above that this may be the case. Weighted least-squares regression analysis is employed, with weights that are proportional to state population in order to reduce heteroskedasticity in the error terms.

We find significant evidence that the growth of managed care is associated with a relative increase in primary care earnings and a decrease in the earnings of many specialists. Table 5–2 reports the relation between managed-care growth and inflation-adjusted changes in median physician income, by specialty grouping and by time period. Table 5–3 summarizes the effect of control variables on the regression estimates.

Between 1985 and 1993, there was significant variation in the rate of growth of primary care physician earnings across managed-care quartiles ($p < .01$). PCP incomes grew more rapidly in states with higher managed-care penetration than in states where managed care was less prevalent. In the states with the highest levels of managed care, average, inflation-adjusted PCP incomes rose at an annual rate of more than 3.3 percent, and there was a cumulative gain in average real earnings equal to $33,000. Primary care physicians in states with the lowest levels of managed-care penetration, however, saw incomes rise only by 1.1 percent annually: $10,400 over the time period in inflation-adjusted dollars.

The pattern of gains for PCPs reversed in 1994. Average PCP earnings fell between 1993 and 1994. Unlike the earlier periods, in which managed-care penetration was associated with higher compensation for PCPs, in 1994 PCPs in high managed-care states saw earnings decline by the largest amounts. PCPs in the markets with lowest levels of penetration reported a modest 1 percent increase in earnings, while PCPs in the markets with highest managed-care penetration, on average, reported that earnings declined by nearly 7 percent. It is interesting to note that among the PCP specialties, general and family practitioners—the least specialized and, generally, lowest compensated specialty group—fared best in recent years. On average, GP/FP earnings rose in 1994 (+1.7 percent), and average increases were reported in all managed-care quartiles. General internists and pediatricians, however, reported sharpest earnings declines in 1994 (−6 percent and −7 percent, respectively). For general internists, the downward trend began in the early 1990s.

While one-year trends should not be overgeneralized, recent evidence for PCPs is consistent with anecdotal claims that plans are showing preferences for using the most general generalists as gatekeepers, and that managed-care contracting may be reducing variation in fee structures—for example, the reimbursements paid for "primary care services" may be quite similar for GP/FPs and general internists, even though historically fees and services may have varied substantially.

Income gains for RAP physicians over the period 1985–1993 also varied across managed-care penetration levels ($p < 0.01$), but in the

TABLE 5-2

ANNUAL GROWTH RATE AND DOLLAR CHANGE IN MEDIAN STATE-LEVEL PHYSICIAN INCOME, BY MANAGED-CARE PENETRATION QUARTILE AND BY SPECIALTY GROUP, 1985–1993 and 1993–1994

Quartile of Managed-Care Penetration, by States	Primary Care		Specialists		RAPs	
	1985–93	1993–94	1985–93	1993–94	1985–93	1993–94
First						
Growth rate (%)	1.11	0.95	1.88	1.55	3.96	–8.30
Change ($)	10,400	1,100	29,500	3,300	70,500	–22,000
Second						
Growth rate (%)	2.30	–1.80	3.91	–5.67	3.11	3.96
Change ($)	22,500	–2,400	66,400	–14,200	54,100	10,100
Third						
Growth rate (%)	2.11	–5.20	3.12	–7.80	1.68	1.30
Change ($)	21,100	–7,300	51,700	–19,000	27,400	2,900
Fourth						
Growth rate (%)	3.37	–6.84	2.18	–10.7	0.60	–6.50
Change ($)	33,400	–9,800	34,500	–23,500	10,400	–13,200
p-value, all quartiles equal	0.01	0.03	0.06	0.04	0.01	0.05

NOTE: Changes in state-level inflation-adjusted average physician income, 1985–1994, by specialty group: cumulative real dollar changes and annual growth rates.
SOURCE: Calculations based on authors' models.

TABLE 5–3
EFFECTS OF SOCIODEMOGRAPHIC CONTROL VARIABLES
ON REGRESSION ESTIMATES FOR PRIMARY CARE,
SUBSPECIALISTS, AND RAPs

	Estimated Signs and Significance of Regression Coefficients					
	Primary care		Subspecialists		RAPS	
Control Variables	*Coef.*	*p-value*	*Coef.*	*p-value*	*Coef.*	*p-value*
Birth rate	934.22	.05	303.44	.54	−758.6	.35
% population under 5	−5083.1	.49	5442.8	.29	−1587.4	.31
% population over 65	275.0	.09	4289.9	.04	10170.5	.06
% nonwhite	−596.3	.09	−6162.2	.17	−5830.6	.10
% uninsured	−550.4	.19	−178.6	.056	−112.9	.97
% urban	1026.6	.02	3386.4	.01	12374.1	.03
Per capita income	3.49	.08	20.25	.08	8.24	.26
% high school graduates	−904.5	.59	−469.1	.69	1343.3	.70
Adjusted R-squared	0.348		0.179		0.451	

SOURCE: Calculations based on authors' model.

opposite direction from that of their primary care colleagues. RAP incomes grew significantly more slowly in states with high managed-care penetration. In the states with the highest levels of managed care, RAP earnings rose by 1 percent per year, or $10,400 from 1985 to 1994. In states with the lowest rates of managed care, RAP incomes grew at a rate of nearly 4 percent, corresponding to a rise in inflation-adjusted income equal to more than $70,000.

In 1994, the pattern generally continued in the middle and higher managed-care markets: RAP earnings fell by more than 6 percent in the top managed-care quartile, grew modestly (1.3 percent) in states in the next highest managed-care stratum, and rose 3 percent in states in the third highest managed-care quartile. Breaking with the pattern of previous years, however, RAPs in the lowest managed-care states reported that average earnings fell by 8 percent (−$22,000).

The 1985–1993 results for medical and surgical specialists are less compelling, and the statistical and economic significance of the differences in income growth across quartiles is much weaker ($p = .09$). Specialist earnings grew the fastest in states characterized by average levels of managed-care penetration. Earnings rose by 1.9 percent annually, or more than $29,000 cumulatively, in the low managed-care markets. Specialists in the highest managed-care states posted real increases in income of $34,000 (2.2 percent annually) between 1985 and 1993, while specialists in the mid-range managed-care markets fared quite well: earnings rose by 3–4 percent in real terms annually, or $51,000–$66,000 over the eight-year period. To the extent that managed care was altering the use of specialist services in this time period, the effect was neither sufficiently large nor sufficiently uniform to be captured in the average, market-level earnings of specialist physicians.

Average specialist earnings fell sharply in 1994: specialists in the highest managed-care markets posted a drop in earnings of almost 11 percent ($23,000), while physicians in the second and third managed-care quartiles saw earnings decline by 5 to 7 percent ($14,000–19,000). Only specialists in the lowest managed-care markets reported modest (1.5 percent) increases in earnings. Still, the 1.5 percent rise in specialty pay in the first quartile was significantly below historic norms. One year is no basis for a trend. In the discussion below we overlay some of the latest evidence on physician compensation to see if earnings changes documented in 1994 presage a significant managed-care–driven decline in the demand for specialty services and specialist pay, or whether other, more transitory factors are at work.

Managed Care and Physician Location

We construct state and specialty-group specific physician-to-population ratios to gauge variations in per capita physician supply. Only nonfederal, patient care physicians are included. Data on physicians' location and self-designated specialty are drawn from the AMA Masterfile (AMA). We recognize that there are trade-offs in using states as our market definition for location decisions. Indeed, if physicians respond to growth in managed care by relocating to less heavily managed-care dominated areas in the same state, then our analysis will not capture adjustments to managed care. As figure 5–1 illustrates, however, there is considerable variation in the levels and growth rates of managed care across states, and this supports a meaningful analysis. Furthermore, there are data problems as one drills down below the state level: moving to finer markets requires one to focus exclusively on urban areas and SMSAs.

State population is based on U.S. Census estimates for the resident population. Population projections compiled by the U.S. Census Bu-

TABLE 5–4

ANNUAL GROWTH RATE OF STATE-LEVEL MANAGED-CARE PENETRATION
AND CHANGES IN PHYSICIAN SUPPLY, BY SPECIALTY GROUP, 1985–1994

Quartile of Managed-Care Penetration, by States	Primary Care	Subspecialists	RAPs
First			
Growth (%)	1.41	2.79	3.22
p-value	.09	.04	.05
Second			
Growth (%)	1.90	3.01	3.28
p-value	.07	.06	.17
Third			
Growth (%)	1.75	2.77	2.46
p-value	.04	.31	.08
Fourth			
Growth (%)	1.33	1.98	2.01
p-value	.23	.10	.05
p-value, all quartiles equal	.09	.05	.01

NOTE: Annualized percentage growth rate, state-level, specialty-specific physician-to-population ratios, 1985–1994; p-values for lowest managed-care quartile test if changes are significantly different from zero; p-values reported for cells in second–fourth quartiles test if results are significantly different from the first quartile.
SOURCE: Calculations based on authors' model.

reau are used to extrapolate the population numbers from the 1980 and 1990 censuses to 1985 and 1993 (U.S. Bureau of the Census). Annualized rates of growth in physicians' per capita incomes are computed at the state level for each of our three physician-specialty groups, yielding a total of 153 observations. Separate, weighted least-squares regressions are estimated for each specialty group. The effect of managed care is measured using indicator variables constructed from the managed-care quartiles, as described above.

Table 5–4 reports regression-adjusted changes in specialty-specific physician supply. Results are broken out by managed-care quartiles and annualized over the period 1985–1994.

There are significant differences across specialty groups and managed-care quartiles, consistent with changes in earnings opportunities. States with the highest levels of managed care (quartile 4) experienced lower growth of subspecialist- and RAP physician-to-population ratios, although only the results for RAPs are statistically significant at conventional levels ($p = .04$). RAP physician-to-population ratios rose 40 percent faster in states in the lowest managed-care growth quartile relative to states experiencing the highest degrees of managed-care growth.

For PCPs, our findings are less clear. Contrary to expectations, there is no compelling evidence that employment opportunities for PCPs have risen in high managed-care areas. States in the middle managed-care quartiles experienced significantly larger increases in primary care physician-to-population ratios than did states in the lowest quartile ($p < .05$). The growth in primary care physicians per capita, however, was lowest for states with the highest levels of managed care. Note, the primary care physician-to-population ratio increased at a slower rate than did the ratios for subspecialists and RAP physicians in all managed-care growth quartiles. This reflects the small pool of primary care physicians entering the work force, which itself may be related to the relatively low earnings of primary care physicians during the time period studied.

Evidence on Specialty Choice

The National Residency Matching Program (NRMP) matches graduating medical school seniors and foreign medical graduates with participating graduate residency training programs. The majority of matches are for programs beginning in the students' first postgraduate year (PGY-1). Some specialty programs, however, do not begin until the second postgraduate year (PGY-2), following a transitional year. The NRMP matches some students simultaneously to PGY-1 transitional positions and selected PGY-2 programs. Postgraduate positions for some medical subspecialties (such as cardiology) are not filled through the match. While some of the unfilled slots are subsequently filled following the match, researchers have historically viewed trends in match data as reflecting medical students' perceptions of the attractiveness of alternative specialties.

Table 5–5 reports the number of PGY-1 and PGY-2 positions, broken down by specialty, that were offered in the NRMP match, and the number (and proportion) that were filled by U.S. medical school graduates for the period 1989 to 1997. For the PGY-1 primary care programs (family practice and pediatrics) we note a general increase in the number of available slots and proportion of positions that are filled. Between 1989 and 1997 the combined number of family practice and pediatrics positions increased by 23.7 percent, and the number of posi-

113

TABLE 5–5
SELECTED SPECIALTY PGY-1 AND PGY-2 POSITIONS OFFERED AND FILLED BY U.S. MEDICAL SCHOOL GRADUATES, 1989–1997

Program	1989 Offered	1989 Filled	1991 Offered	1991 Filled	1993 Offered	1993 Filled	1994 Offered	1994 Filled	1995 Offered	1995 Filled	1996 Offered	1996 Filled	1997 Offered	1997 Filled
Primary care: PGY-1														
Family practice	2,456	1,469 (59.8)	2,487	1,385 (55.7)	2,589	1,636 (63.2)	2,774	1,850 (66.7)	2,941	2,082 (70.8)	3,137	2,277 (72.6)	3,262	2,340 (71.7)
Pediatrics	2,012	1,227 (61.0)	2,009	1,298 (64.6)	2,008	1,339 (66.7)	2,017	1,404 (69.6)	2,029	1,465 (72.9)	2,017	1,547 (76.7)	2,019	1,650 (79.0)
Specialties: PGY-1														
Surgical specialty	553	484 (87.6)	647	555 (85.8)	708	608 (85.9)	715	576 (80.6)	706	617 (87.4)	708	599 (84.6)	736	654 (88.9)
All RAPs	1,112	715 (64.3)	1,226	858 (70.0)	1,259	818 (65.0)	1,182	747 (63.2)	1,167	693 (59.4)	1,118	468 (41.9)	874	304 (34.8)
Anesthesiology only	293	200 (68.4)	329	250 (76.1)	325	199 (61.2)	297	163 (54.9)	251	93 (37.1)	348	43 (17.3)	317	80 (25.2)
Support specialties: PGY-1 + PGY-2														
All RAPs	2,285	1,568 (68.6)	2,630	1,867 (71.0)	2,811	1,807 (64.3)	2,642	1,635 (61.9)	2,619	1,361 (52.0)	2,540	1,140 (44.9)	2,243	864 (38.5)
Anesthesiology only	1,053	737 (70.0)	1,292	944 (73.1)	1,419	832 (58.6)	1,319	711 (53.9)	1,153	442 (38.3)	960	168 (17.5)	994	252 (25.4)

NOTE: Numbers in parentheses are the percentages of slots filled.
SOURCE: Authors' calculations based on National Residency Match Program data.

114

tions filled increased by 48 percent.[2]

We find modest evidence of an increase in the attractiveness of surgical specialty training in the early part of our study period, followed by stable numbers of positions and matches, but showing new growth in the latest year. Between 1989 and 1993, positions increased by 28 percent, from 553 to 708, with little change in the proportion of positions filled. From 1993 to 1996, both the number of residency positions available and the number filled remained relatively constant. In 1997, there was a 4 percent increase in specialty surgery slots and more than a 9 percent rise in the number of new physicians electing to take them.

We present information on both PGY-1 positions alone and for PGY-1 and PGY-2 positions combined for RAP programs, and for programs in anesthesiology in particular. Trends are similar. We focus here on combined PGY-1 and PGY-2 numbers. The number of slots in PGY-1 and PGY-2 RAP programs rose by 11 percent between 1989 and 1996, peaking in 1993. Between 1996 and 1997, the combined available supply of slots shrank by 12 percent, with most of the reductions coming in programs in diagnostic radiology. There have been sharp changes in the demand for slots as well. The number of U.S. medical school graduates matched with these positions fell by more than 38 percentage points between 1989 and 1996: the share of positions filled fell from roughly 70 percent in 1989–1991 to under 50 percent in 1996. Even with the reduction in slots, the proportion filled fell further in 1997—to 864 graduates matched with RAP programs in 1997, down from 1,140 in 1996. Virtually all the decline was accounted for by positions in anesthesiology up to 1996: filled anesthesiology positions totaled 1,419 in 1993, but only 960 in 1996. In 1997 retrenchment in radiology drove the aggregate results.

Discussion

We have presented economic evidence that suggests that the growth of managed care has had substantial and widespread effects in the physician marketplace. Over much of the period the incomes of primary care physicians grew most rapidly, and the incomes of RAP physicians least rapidly, in markets characterized by high managed-care penetration. The incomes of medical and surgical subspecialists also lagged in markets with the highest managed care, although the results for the

---

2. We do not track positions in internal medicine, since many of the physicians who complete internal medicine go on to specialty residency and fellowship programs.

specialist group are less significant both economically and statistically. These findings suggest that the spread of managed care is significantly altering the relative compensation and employment of primary care and specialist physicians.

Since we completed this study the AMA has released new survey data. The 1995 income data suggest that, for some specialties, earnings rebounded in 1995. We do not have access to these data for detailed analysis, but we can reexamine the trends we have identified in light of the newly published statistics (American Medical News 1997; Gonzalez 1997). While the AMA notes that "[nominal] physician earnings climbed 7 percent in 1995," adjusting for inflation, the two-year trend still shows a loss in earnings power for the average physician. Looking across specialties, between 1993 and 1995 real earnings fell by more than 4.5 percent for medical and surgical specialists, declined more than 8 percent for RAPs, but rose 8.7 percent for primary care physicians. In general, the specialty trends are consistent with our work. Primary care is clearly in a flux. Earnings have been volatile and future trends are unclear.[3]

Over time physicians will tend to migrate to those areas that offer superior compensation and working conditions. Our findings for RAP physicians are consistent with this prediction. States with the highest managed-care growth had the lowest increases in RAP physician-to-population ratios. A similar pattern of growth was documented for the subspecialist group, although results were not statistically significant. Our failure to document managed-care related patterns in specialist location is congruous with our lack of strong findings that managed care has altered specialist earnings.

While earnings of PCPs were positively linked to managed-care penetration, we do not find corresponding evidence that the numbers of PCPs have risen in the strongest managed-care markets. There are at least two potential explanations. First, it is possible that managed-care organizations were attracted to areas that already had high numbers of primary care physicians, so that even though competing managed-care organizations bid up incomes, the need for additional

---

3. Care must be exercised when comparing the published AMA statistics with the income numbers reported in this chapter. First, our specialty categories are not identical with the definitions used in AMA publications. Second, we have adjusted the net income numbers so that deferred income is treated identically in all years of our time series. There were changes in the SMS survey that affected reporting of physicians' deferred compensation in 1994 and 1995. The AMA unadjusted trends are more volatile than our corrected income series.

primary care physicians was small and hence growth rates were low. Dranove, Simon, and White (1997) have shown that managed-care penetration has been higher in markets with greater competition among providers. The results in this chapter suggest the need to explore the extent to which physician supply has affected managed-care penetration and growth.

Second, it is possible that there are negative, nonpecuniary attributes associated with delivering primary care in a managed-care environment (Chawla, Kletke, and Emmons, 1995). This would raise earnings but not employment opportunities. Finally, supply may be adjusting on other margins: incumbent PCPs may be working more hours or devoting a larger proportion of the practice day to delivering primary care services. In other work, we have found evidence that physicians who have contracts with managed-care organizations narrow their scope of practice: PCPs increase the share of their time devoted to primary care, while specialists devote more time to specialty care (Simon et al. 1997).

Finally, evidence from the National Residency Match Programs indicates that residency programs are opening more positions in primary care and that a growing number of young physicians are electing to fill them. At the same time, programs are reducing the number of positions in selected specialties, and fewer young physicians are electing to fill them.

Taken together, our results suggest that there is more to managed care than sorting patients; results are consistent with substantial market-level effects on the relative incomes of primary care and specialty physicians and on specialists per capita. Managed care has had the largest effect on the services of hospital-based physicians—and only modest changes in the use and compensation of medical and surgical specialists. Finally, while PCP earnings have risen, there is less compelling evidence that there has been an increase in the number of physicians employed in high managed-care markets. It remains to be seen if this is evidence of a short-run imbalance or longer-run requirements.

Evidence from the specialty choices of new medical graduates indicates that young physicians are cognizant of shifts in compensation and expect patterns to persist. In light of the relatively recent nature of changes in physician earnings, the documented changes in supply and specialty choice are quite remarkable. Looking forward, continuation of current trends would translate into substantial changes in the relative numbers of primary care and specialist physicians. Combined with other recent evidence on physician behavior (Hillman et al. 1989), they suggest that public policy makers have to take into account the fact that significant market adjustments are already underway in the physician marketplace.

References

The AMCRA Foundation Managed Health Care Overview. 1995. Washington, D.C.

American Medical Association. Various years. *Physician Characteristics and Distribution in the U.S.* Chicago, Ill.

Anders, G. 1995. "Numb and Number: Once a Hot Specialty, Anesthesiology Cools as Insurers Scale Back." *Wall Street Journal,* March 17, p. 1.

Arnould, R., et al. 1984. "Do HMOs Produce Specific Services More Efficiently?" *Inquiry* 21:243–53.

Chawla, A. J., P. R. Kletke, and D. W. Emmons. 1995. "Specialty Satisfaction among Young Physicians: Implications for Primary Care." American Medical Association manuscript, June.

Congressional Budget Office. 1994. "Effects of Managed Care: An Update," April.

Dial, T., S. Palsbo, C. Bergsten, J. Gabel, and J. Weiner. 1995. "Clinical Staffing in Staff and Group-Model HMOs." *Health Affairs* 14(2):168–80.

Dranove, David, Carol Simon, and William White. 1997. "Determinants of Managed Care Penetration." *Journal of Health Economics,* forthcoming.

Eisenberg, J. 1994. "If Trickle-Down Physician Workforce Policy Failed, Is the Choice Now between the Market and Government Regulation?" *Inquiry* 31(3):241–49.

Emmons, D., and C. Simon. 1996. "Managed Care: Evolving Contracting Patterns." *Socioeconomic Characteristics of Medical Practice.* Chicago: American Medical Association.

Franks, P., C. Clancy, and P. Nutting. 1992. "Gatekeeping Revisited—Protecting Patients from Overtreatment." *New England Journal of Medicine* 327:424–29.

Gamliel, S., et al. 1995. "Managed Care on the March: Will Physicians Meet the Challenge?" *Health Affairs* (Summer):131–43.

Gaynor, M. 1994. "Issues in the Industrial Organization of the Market for Physician Services." *Journal of Economics and Management Strategy* 3(1):211–55.

Goldman, D. 1995. "Managed Care as a Public Cost-Containment Mechanism." *RAND Journal of Economics* 26(2):277–95.

Gonzalez, M. (ed). 1997. *Socioeconomic Characteristics of Medical Practice, 1996.* Chicago: American Medical Association.

Grumbach, K., and P. Lee. 1991. "How Many Physicians Can We Afford?" *JAMA* 265:2369–72.

Hart, L. G., E. Wagner, S. Pirzada, A. F. Nelson, and R. Rosenblatt. 1997. "Physician Staffing Ratios in Staff-Model HMOs: A Cautionary Tale." *Health Affairs* 16(1):55–70.

Hellinger, F. 1995. "Selection Bias in HMOs and PPOs: A Review of the Evidence." *Inquiry* 32:135–42.

Hillman, A., M. Pauly, and J. Kerstein. 1989. "How Do Financial Incentives Affect Physicians' Clinical Decisions and the Financial Performance of Health Maintenance Organizations?" *New England Journal of Medicine* 321:86–92.

Kindig, D., J. Cultice, and F. Mullan. 1993. "The Elusive Generalist Physician; Can We Reach a 50% Goal?" *JAMA* 270:1069–73.

Kronick, R., et al. 1993. "The Marketplace in Health Care Reform: The Demographic Limitations of Managed Competition." *New England Journal of Medicine* 328:148–52.

Luft, H. 1991. *Health Maintenance Organizations: Dimensions of Performance.* New York: Wiley.

Manning, W., et al. 1984. "A Controlled Trial of the Effect of a Prepaid Group Practice on Use of Services." *New England Journal of Medicine* 310:1505–10.

Marder, W., P. Kletke, A. Silberger, and R. Wilke. 1988. *Physician Supply and Utilization by Specialty: Trends and Projections.* Chicago: American Medical Association.

McGuire, T., and M. Pauly. 1991. "Physician Response to Fee Changes with Multiple Payers." *Journal of Health Economics* 10:385–412.

McKay, N. 1990. "The Economic Determinants of Specialty Choice by Medical Residents." *Journal of Health Economics* 9:335–57.

Moore, G. 1994. "Will the Power of the Marketplace Produce the Workforce We Need?" *Inquiry* 31(3):276–82.

Morgan, W. 1994. "HMO Trend Squeezes Big-Fee Medical Specialists." *Washington Post,* August 17.

Page, L. 1994. "Early Signs of a Shakeout." *American Medical News* 37(37):1.

Reinhardt, U. 1994. "Planning the Nation's Health Workforce: Let the Market Do It." *Inquiry* 31(3):250–63.

Rosenthal, E. 1995. "Young Doctors Find That Jobs in Specialties Are Harder to Get." *New York Times* 144(50), April 16.

Rosenthal, Michael P., et al. 1994. "Influence of Income, Hours Worked, and Loan Repayment on Medical Students' Decision to Pursue a Primary Care Career." *JAMA* 271(12):914–17, March 23/30.

Schroeder, S. 1994. "Managing the U.S. Health Care Workforce: Creating Policy amidst Uncertainty." *Inquiry* 31(3):266–75.

Simon, Carol J., and Patricia Born. 1996. "Physician Earnings in a Changing Managed Care Environment." *Health Affairs* 15(3):124–33.

Simon, Carol J., William D. White, Phillip Kletke, and Sandra Gamliel. 1997. "Physician Provision of Primary Care Services: Does Managed Care Matter?" *Health Affairs* 16(6):89–98.

U.S. Bureau of the Census. 1992. "Current Population Reports." Series P-25, nos. 1058, 1045 and 1024. Washington, D.C.: Government Printing Office.

Wennberg, J., D. Goodman, R. Nease, and R. Keller. 1993. "Finding Equilibrium in U.S. Physician Supply." *Health Affairs* 12(2):89–103.

6
Market Definition in Antitrust Analysis and Applications to Health Care

David Dranove

Market definition is a cornerstone of antitrust analysis. In an antitrust claim, the plaintiff (either a government agency or a private claimant) alleges that one or more firms have engaged in anticompetitive activity in violation of the Sherman Act or some other antitrust statute. To prosecute its claim successfully, the plaintiff must usually show that the defendant(s) possesses market power, either alone or when acting in concert. To do so, the plaintiff must identify a "relevant" product and geographic market. The relevant market would include those competitors who could provide consumers with alternatives if the defendant should raise prices or otherwise injure consumers.[1]

Very often, judicial rulings in antitrust cases turn on whether the courts accept the plaintiff's or the defense's market definition.[2] A hospital merger in Rockford, Illinois, for example, was denied when the court held to a narrow market definition, whereas a merger under seemingly similar circumstances in Roanoke, Virginia, was approved when a different court accepted a broader market definition.[3] This chapter discusses principles of market definition and current market definition strategies in health care antitrust cases. I argue that current

Thanks go out to William White, Mark Satterthwaite, Martin Gaynor, Michael Morrisey, and an anonymous reviewer who provided valuable insights.

1. While consumer injury may take many forms, such as in tying arrangements that force consumers to purchase products that they would prefer not to purchase, I will refer mainly to price increases. This is merely for convenience, not because price increases are the only antitrust concern in health care.

2. An important recent exception is Federal Trade Commission v. Butterworth Health Corporation and Blodgett Memorial Medical Center, in which the judge accepted the FTC market definition but upheld the merger.

3. For further discussion of these cases see Allen et al. (1989).

strategies, which are based on traditional models of competition, may lead to an underestimation of antitrust risks in health care. Strategies for market definition that recognize emerging health care institutions are more appropriate and may identify greater risks.

Some Basics of Market Definition

The main purpose of market definition in antitrust analysis is to determine if the defendant has sufficient market power to raise prices. If the court finds that other firms constrain the ability of the defendant to raise prices, then it will usually presume that any anticompetitive actions by the defendants would not succeed, because consumers would take their business elsewhere. In this case, the court would not intervene in the defendant's business practices.

If the aim of the court is to determine if the defendant faces the discipline of market competition, then market definition for antitrust analysis should seek to identify other firms that may *constrain* the defendant's actions. To crystallize the idea of market constraints, consider the competition faced by a seller of local telephone exchange services, such as NYNEX or Ameritech. Currently, each local exchange service has a government-sanctioned monopoly in the region it serves. If, say, Ameritech were to raise prices for local calls in its market by 20 percent, consumers in the upper Midwest (Ameritech's service area) would have little choice but to pay the higher price or cut back on local calls.[4] The reason is that no other firms offer local exchange service and thereby constrain Ameritech. Consider instead the competition faced by a long-distance carrier such as AT&T. If it were to raise its price for long-distance calls by 20 percent, some customers might remain loyal to it, but many others would switch to other carriers such as MCI and Sprint. Hence, MCI and Sprint constrain AT&T.

The most direct way to determine if a firm is constrained by others is to determine *own-price* and *cross-price elasticities* of demand. A firm's own-price elasticity of demand is the percentage change in its sales quantity in response to a 1 percent change in its price. The cross-price elasticity of demand between firms X and Y is the percentage change in Y's sales quantity in response to a 1 percent change in firm X's price. The cross-price elasticity is intuitively appealing because it identifies firms that may constrain each other. But one cannot readily determine from cross-price elasticities whether a firm can profitably sustain a price increase. Suppose, for example, that the cross-price elasticity of

---

4. Electronic mail might be an acceptable substitute for some consumers at some times.

demand between firms X and Y is large in magnitude, but firm Y is relatively small compared with firm X. Then firm X may raise its price and lose very few sales, even while firm Y enjoys a large increase in its sales (in percentage terms).

The own-price elasticity directly indicates whether a firm or group of firms may profitably sustain a price increase.[5] Of course, a monopolist that prices correctly will already have raised its price to the point where further increases are unprofitable. In this case, it may be difficult to infer monopoly power from the own-price elasticity. The measure may be more useful when computed for hypothetical combinations of firms. These firms may face elastic demand because of the constraints they impose on each other. But a merger would allow them to coordinate pricing. In this case, the (hypothetical) own-price elasticity facing the combination of firms would indicate if they faced competition from other firms.

To illustrate how the own-price elasticity may be used to examine hypothetical combinations, suppose that Miller and Budweiser Breweries were to consolidate into a single beer retailing giant. Currently, Miller and Bud may face large own-price elasticities because of competition from each other. If they were to consolidate, the own-price elasticity facing "Budmiller" might be rather small, particularly if consumers believe that there are no viable alternatives to Bud and Miller. In this case, the combined Budmiller might find it profitable to raise price substantially. One suspects that in this particular case, the own-price elasticity facing Budmiller would still be fairly large, with other brewers such as Coors serving to constrain price increases.

Economists use an empirical methodology called "residual demand curve" estimation to compute own-price elasticities for hypothetical combinations of firms.[6] Economists within the antitrust agencies have argued that residual demand curve analysis is the preferred method for market definition—especially for merger analysis—as it provides direct evidence on whether hypothetical combinations of firms can profitably raise prices. But the data requirements for residual demand curve analysis can be severe, especially in health care markets. The analyst must have data on prices, costs, and instruments for costs (that is, variables that cause costs to differ across firms but are unrelated to demand). It is often difficult to get good price data in health care. Even with the benefits of the discovery process in an anti-

---

5. One would also need information about the present price level, P, and marginal cost, MC. If the own-elasticity is smaller in magnitude than the present price cost margin ($[P - MC]/P$), then the firm can prosper by raising prices.

6. For an overview of this methodology, see Bresnahan (1989).

trust proceeding, price data can be complex because of product differentiation and variations in payment methods across insurers. It may be even more difficult to obtain good instruments for costs. In most published residual demand curve studies, sellers are geographically separated, and researchers can use variations in local input costs as identifiers of variations in production costs. But health care markets are local, and competing sellers generally face similar cost conditions within their local markets. Thus, variations in input costs across competitors will be minimal.[7]

Given data limitations, one rarely sees elasticity estimates in health care antitrust cases.[8] Instead, economists rely on more intuitive approaches to market definition, which I describe below. These approaches may be divided into those used for defining product markets and those used for defining geographic markets.

Product Market Definition

Intuitively, products are in the same product market if they share the same *product performance characteristics* and the same *occasions for use*. Product performance characteristics may be thought of as the underlying hedonic characteristics of the product. Hence, WebTV and personal computers may be in the same product market, at least for some consumers, because they both provide Internet access. Occasions for use of seemingly similar products may differ; for example, orange juice is almost exclusively a breakfast drink, but orange soda is not.

Defining a product market in health care usually follows these intuitive ideas. Courts have accepted product market definitions such as the "market for acute inpatient services" or the "market for professional radiology services." Such definitions are based largely on assertions that hospitals or radiologists provide services not normally provided by other classes of providers. In the case of hospitals, this is no doubt true. Despite the growth of outpatient care, many services are provided almost exclusively by hospitals, including most sophisticated surgical procedures such as total hip replacements and coronary artery bypass grafts. An important class of "hospital-only" services is mater-

---

7. Different sellers may have different input costs, but this could reflect quality differences. The idea is that it is often impossible to identify exogenous sources of cost differences.

8. To my knowledge, the only elasticity estimates that have been introduced were based on surveys in which consumers were asked how their consumption would change if prices changed. It is not clear whether such surveys provide an accurate gauge of actual behavior.

nity, newborn, and neonatal care. Not only do many hospitals rely on these services for substantial revenues, but also it is common for only a subset of hospitals in a given geographic market to offer them. Thus, one may find market power in the market for maternity (or, especially, neonatology) services, even in markets where there is otherwise substantial competition among hospitals.[9]

Regardless of whether the market is defined as "the market for acute inpatient services" or "the market for neonatology services," the implicit assumption is that price is determined by the interaction between the providers of such services and the patients consuming them. But as managed care has come to dominate many markets, price appears to be set by the interactions of payers and providers rather than by the interaction of patients and providers. Prices are set in what payers and providers call the "market for managed-care contracts."

Without a doubt, managed care has fundamentally changed the way that providers set prices. A critical question for antitrust is whether the nature of market constraints, and the resulting market definition, differs when competition is payer driven. I believe that it does.

Payer-driven Competition and Product Market Definition. Managed-care payers assemble networks of providers that they market to employers and their employees. Under payer-driven competition, providers compete to be part of provider networks. Insurers assemble these networks and offer them to employers and their employees as part of managed-care plans. Hence, when consumers sign up for a managed-care plan they are, in essence, selecting a provider network. If a desired provider is not part of that network, the consumer must forgo the use of that provider for the entire year, unless they are willing to pay the full price.[10] This implies that pricing is determined by two factors: (1) competition among hospitals to enter networks; and (2) to the extent that hospitals have consolidated into chains, the number of local networks. The two issues are intertwined, as mergers of individual hospitals affect both the formation of networks and the number of viable

---

9. In an antitrust case that I recently worked on, the evidence showed that neonatology patients were far less likely to be admitted to a distant hospital than were average patients.

10. Even if managed-care plans offer some coverage for out-of-plan use, that coverage is often limited. Not only must the patient pay a higher copayment (typically 30 percent), but the patient may be responsible for the difference between the provider's charge and the lower amount that the insurer deems is reasonable. This difference may dwarf the 30 percent copayment.

networks. In the next section, I discuss why these considerations may radically alter geographic market definition. They may also affect the definition of the product market, as I now discuss.

In most of the hospital antitrust cases that I have studied, few efforts have been made to identify "submarkets" of general hospitals—for example, neonatology providers—that may constitute a distinct market for certain services. The need to identify product submarkets emerges in a different way when we consider competition to be included in managed-care contracts.

I have reviewed the structure of managed-care contracts in several metropolitan areas. Those contracts almost always include at least one local tertiary care hospital. Several possible reasons account for why managed-care contracts seem always to include at least one such institution. One obvious reason is that tertiary care hospitals may be the only sellers of certain services. In this case, those hospitals serve a distinct product market, albeit one that is limited in size. Interestingly, included among these "unique" services are transplants and open heart surgery, for which the geographic market may be very large. (Some managed-care purchasers "carve out" these specialized services and require patients to travel out of town to receive them.)

If we ignore the specialized services such as transplants, managed-care purchasers include at least one tertiary care hospital for other reasons, creating a "submarket" of such hospitals. One reason why managed-care contracts include tertiary care hospitals may be to signal overall quality. Because consumers have difficulty in determining the quality of hospitals, they may well be suspicious of the motives of some managed-care organizations when they assemble networks, given the occasional bad publicity received by managed-care payers. Surely those suspicions would be heightened if the network excluded those hospitals with the best reputation for quality, generally tertiary care hospitals. In this case, such hospitals create an externality for the managed-care payer by providing a patina of quality.

Another reason why tertiary care hospitals may be important to managed-care payers and therefore constitute a product submarket stems from what Dranove and White (1996) call "option demand." When individuals sign up for a managed-care plan, they are uncertain about their future medical needs. If they believe that they have even a small chance of requiring the quality of care often available only at tertiary care hospitals, they may be willing to pay a premium to ensure such access. Thus, they value having the option of access to that kind of hospital; I call this premium an "access fee." The idea that providers may extract an access fee is taken up again when I discuss geographic market power.

While tertiary care hospitals may provide value to managed-care payers and their subscribers, that value may be competed away in markets with several. But if there is only one, or there is more than one but they interact in ways that do not drive prices down to costs, the hospital(s) could extract much of this value. Barro and Cutler (1997), for example, conjecture that the merger of Massachusetts General Hospital and Brigham and Women's Hospital created a "new institution so prestigious that most insurers virtually cannot afford not to contract with it." This enhanced prestige has thus enabled the merged hospitals to prosper.

The claim that tertiary care hospitals may represent a unique product submarket is not inconsistent with Zwanziger and Meirowitz's finding elsewhere in this book that *teaching* (as opposed to tertiary care) hospitals are less likely to be included in contracts. Perhaps managed-care payers want only one teaching or tertiary care hospital, so that the probability that others will be added to the network is low. In contrast, in older research, Feldman and others (1990) find that teaching hospitals are more likely to be included in networks. Inclusion at a higher price may have had a cost, however. They find that enrollees in at least some forms of managed care were less likely to go to the higher-priced teaching hospitals.

In some markets, tertiary care hospitals have actively sought to increase the perceived value of access by making substantial investments to establish brand awareness. One of the largest provider advertisers in the Chicago market is the University of Chicago Hospitals and Clinics (UCHC), which boasts of its cutting-edge medical care. Its advertisements run heavily during the late fall, at a time when many employees are selecting their health plans under open enrollment. The ads are probably intended to increase the demand for managed-care plans that include UCHC, thereby enabling UCHC to increase its prices. (Of course, other tertiary care hospitals have run similar promotions, and if consumers view them as close substitutes for UCHC, prices will be constrained.)

Retail Pharmacy. The previous discussion makes two points. The first point—that local sellers may possess market power—pertains specifically to payer-driven competition. The second point is more general: the resolution of market definition issues should depend on the institutions under study. It is essential to understand the process that generates prices before determining which competitors' interactions determine prices. In many markets, prices are determined by complex interactions between buyers and sellers whose outcomes may or may not be well met by simple textbook models of competition. The retail pharmacy market provides a good example of this.

A number of retail pharmacies have merged in recent years. One proposed merger—between Rite-Aid and Revco—was withdrawn after a challenge by the Federal Trade Commission. In mergers such as these, it may be necessary to determine whether other retail pharmacies (or any other firms, for that matter) constrain the ability of the merging pharmacies to raise prices. The managed-care payers in the retail pharmacy market are called pharmacy benefits managers, or PBMs. They contract with a subset of all the retail pharmacies in an area. Patients whose managed-care plans contract with a particular PBM will be covered for prescription drug costs only if they obtain them from a contracting pharmacy. The contracting pharmacy agrees to dispense drugs at a discount from its normal rate.

At the time of the proposed merger, Rite-Aid and Revco were two of the largest pharmacy chains in the United States. Moreover, they were the two largest chains in a number of metropolitan areas in which they both competed. While one might consider each individual pharmacy to be in a unique market, facing unique competitive environments, there were compelling reasons to view the geographic market as the metro area. The most important reason was that the PBMs sold their pharmacy networks to employers, who generally had to accept or reject the network in its entirety. Thus, a relevant question for antitrust analysis was whether the merger limited the ability of PBMs to assemble competing viable pharmacy networks within an employer's region. Specifically, if a viable network would have to include either Rite-Aid or Revco, then the merger would effectively reduce the number of competitors from two to one. Metro areas were used as a reasonable proxy for the region from which most employers attract employees.

PBMs could conceivably have turned to other pharmacies to assemble alternative networks, however. Potential network pharmacies included other chains (for example, CVS), pharmacies operated by mass merchandisers (for example, Wal-Mart), mail-order pharmacies (for example, Medco), and independent pharmacies. Evidence suggested, however, that networks usually formed around anchor pharmacy chains—large, well-known chains with many locations within the metro area. One reason offered was that consumers are more willing to accept limitations on pharmacy choice if the network includes a large, easy-to-find pharmacy chain.

Another reason is that larger chains often have lower costs, so that PBMs could reduce prices by playing the large chains off against each other. Indeed, once the PBM established a low price from one anchor, it often used this as the basis for making a take-it-or-leave-it offer to other, smaller chains. In this way, the competition between the large chains established the price paid to all pharmacies. If this analysis is correct, then PBMs would surely benefit from the presence of independent Rite-Aid and Revco chains in those metro areas where they were both large enough to serve as anchors. Had they merged, they might have been the only viable anchor and could have raised prices.

Geographic Market Definition

The standard tool for determining the geographic extent of health care markets is the Elzinga-Hogarty test. Hogarty and Elzinga (1973) proposed their test in conjunction with an analysis of the geographic extent of coal markets. They examined the flow of coal into and out of candidate markets and argued that a geographic market for coal is well defined if imports and exports are small. The E-H test suggests that imports are small if they represent less than 10–25 percent of the total sales to customers in the market and that exports are small if they represent less than 10–25 percent of production by sellers in the market. Although Hogarty and Elzinga discuss product flows, the approach is easily adaptable to customer flows in the case of services markets.

The E-H test is attractive for several reasons. First, it seems to capture the substitution patterns of buyers both in and out of the potential market. If there are substantial customer outflows, then it stands to reason that consumers consider firms outside the candidate market to be viable alternatives. Substantial inflows would indicate that firms in the candidate market do much of their business with consumers outside the area and thus may be competing for those consumers with sellers outside the area. In either case, the candidate market would seem to be too small. The second attraction of the E-H test—at least in health care—is that it is fairly easy to employ, particularly with the types of data on patient flows available from Medicare and many state health agencies.

Because of its appeal, many health care antitrust cases rely on the E-H test for geographic market definition. But antitrust economists such as Werden (1992) have pointed out that there is no necessary connection between patient flows and the degree to which local sellers may raise prices. If products are homogeneous and transportation costs are nil, for example, then buyers and sellers will interact locally, and both imports and exports will be nonexistent. Yet if sellers raised prices by only a tiny amount, imports would increase substantially. In this case, the E-H test might substantially underestimate potential competition and lead to a misleadingly small geographic market.

While this criticism of the E-H test may be of some concern in health care applications, there is another problem with E-H that may cause markets to be defined too broadly. The test implicitly assumes that products and services are homogeneous, except for transportation costs. But health care goods and services tend to be differentiated on a number of dimensions that reflect patients' idiosyncratic preferences for particular providers. Such preferences may be based on medical factors such as bedside manner, practice style, or even cultural factors such as language or ethnicity. Patients may also develop those preferences if they have favorable experiences with one provider and are unwilling to switch to another provider in whom they have less confidence. The important implication for the E-H test is that patients with idiosyncratic preferences for one or more local sellers will not readily switch to sellers in other areas merely because of a slight imbalance in prices.

To some extent, observed inflows and outflows reflect idiosyncrasies whereby patients travel out of their local community to seek care elsewhere, even though seemingly similar providers are located nearby. Several types of idiosyncrasies could generate patient flows:

- An individual lives in town A but works in town B. That person becomes seriously ill while at work and is admitted to a hospital in town B. That person does not necessarily consider hospitals in the two towns to be substitutes nor would price reduction by hospitals in town A necessarily have changed the admission decision.

- Along the same lines, an individual lives in town A but is visiting or vacationing in town B; that person becomes ill while in town B. Or an individual lives part of the year in town B but lists a permanent residence in town A.

- An individual lives in town A but has developed a strong relationship with a physician who admits patients to hospitals in town B. As with the previous examples, a change in the relative prices of hospitals in towns A and B may have no influence on this patient's admission decision.

The presence of idiosyncratic travel implies that we would likely observe some patient travel even if sellers in different markets do not constrain each other's pricing at all. In particular, the above examples suggest that we would likely observe nontrivial flows from small towns to larger cities. Individuals are more likely to work in or visit the larger cities. Moreover, there are more likely to be specialists in large cities to whom patients travel for treatment of complex problems. In most of the E-H analyses that I have seen, the flows are much larger into large cities (from smaller surrounding towns) than out of large cities. Such flows into cities would not necessarily imply that the hospitals in large cities are constrained by the hospitals in smaller towns. Suppose that patients travel for the reasons given above. Then, if big city hospitals were to raise prices in lockstep, most of their out-of-town patients might well continue to use them, as their reasons for doing so in the first place may have had nothing to do with price.[11]

Another weakness of the E-H test that, to my knowledge, has not received much attention is the implicit assumption that sellers cannot price discriminate. Specifically, the logic of the E-H analysis holds that if hospitals sell to consumers outside the candidate market, they must charge the same price as they do to local consumers. This is a critical assumption, because it implies that if local sellers raise their prices to exploit their alleged market power in their local market, they may lose valuable business from consumers who reside outside the local market. (These consumers now turn to their own local sellers.) This is supposed to limit the ability of sellers to raise prices when exports (that is, inflows) are high. If sellers can price discriminate, this limit does not exist. They can raise local prices while suppressing prices charged to more distant customers. In the case of health care markets, some price discrimination appears possible, especially when providers are negotiating with managed-care companies that may have different rates of penetration in different areas. When price discrimination is possible, local market power is enhanced.

A Managed-Care Environment

The E-H methodology implicitly assumes that patients will discipline high-priced hospitals by taking their "business" elsewhere. Until the past decade or so, it was the case that patients (and their physicians) were largely responsible for selecting hospitals. It might seem reasonable to apply the E-H methodology, which specifically examines patient flows, under such *patient-driven competition*. If patients traveled from one town to another to receive hospital care, it might be reasonable to conclude that hospitals in both towns constrained one another and belonged in the same geographic market. But a casual analysis of historical pricing data indicates that such a conclusion would have been premature. Moreover, there has been a switch to payer-driven competition, calling into question the reliance on E-H methods that focus on patient decision making. I address these points in turn below.

I will first consider the potentially misleading conclusions of the E-H approach under patient-driven competition. Consider a typical

---

11. The argument may be symmetric to small town hospitals, providing that patients leave small towns for reasons other than price.

metropolitan area around 1980. If one obtained data on patient travel for that period, one would observe substantial intramarket travel, from suburbs to downtown, from suburb to suburb, and the like. It would not be uncommon, for example, for 50 percent or more of the residents of one suburb to shun their local hospital for another within that metro area. A standard E-H approach would lead one to conclude that each hospital in the metro area competed, directly or indirectly, with each other hospital. The number of competitors in many metro areas would therefore be quite large—Chicago would have nearly eighty competitors, for example. But in spite of the seemingly large number of competitors, hospitals typically set prices well above marginal costs and may have set prices even higher had they not been concerned about nonprofit status.[12] In other words, the many competitors identified by the E-H approach failed to constrain prices.

The failure of competing hospitals to constrain prices is not a problem with the E-H approach per se. Rather, the problem lies with traditional antitrust methods as applied willy-nilly to health care markets under patient-driven competition. Traditional methods assume that the presence of many competitors will drive prices toward costs. But there remains little consensus among health care economists on the mechanisms that constrained provider pricing—and the role of competition—under patient-driven competition. Nonprofit hospitals were certainly constrained by ethical concerns or perhaps fear of losing nonprofit status. But the exact nature of these constraints remains unknown.

Nowadays, health care providers must compete for contracts with managed-care payers. According to a general consensus, payer-driven competition has introduced price pressure into health care markets, as reflected in moderating if not declining provider prices. But the mechanisms used by payers to assemble networks do not resemble those used by individual patients to select providers. Thus, the antitrust tools used to define geographic markets when patients select providers may generate misleading conclusions about the scope of geographic markets when payers select providers.

When assembling managed-care networks, payers typically attempt to provide enrollees with broad geographic coverage for several reasons.[13] When consumers sign up for a managed-care plan, they are, in essence, selecting a provider network. They effectively forgo the use

---

12. For a discussion of whether and how nonprofits exploit market power see *Who Profits from the Not-for-Profit Hospital* (1989).

13. For example, many employers place explicit geographic distribution requirements in their solicitations for managed-care networks.

of providers outside the network. Consumers may value access to a local provider, even if they would not use that provider for all their health care needs and may travel for some of their care. In effect, consumers have an "option value" for the ability to access a local hospital. The value of local access may turn out to be very high, for example, if the patient develops a chronic health problem or if the nearby relatives are unable to travel at the time of the illness. Hence, the option value of local access may be substantial.

But a managed-care plan may offer a network that does not feature broad geographic coverage of providers. Because consumers may value local access highly, someone residing in an area without a contracting provider may be reluctant to sign up for the plan. That individual may instead select another insurer whose network includes a local provider. Because consumers value local access, insurers have an incentive to contract with local providers.

If a locality contains several providers, managed-care plans may play one off against the other to obtain local access at a low cost. If all the providers in a local area were to merge, however, then the managed-care plan would have no choice but to pay a higher price to the merged entity to ensure local access. In this way, the merged entity exploits market power. Local patients, of course, may still travel for some of their care, even as they express their demand for local access. Thus, there is no inconsistency among occasional patient travel, a strong desire for local access, and an incentive for insurers to contract with local providers.

To summarize, traditional antitrust analysis has employed the E-H technique to identify competitors. That technique is problematic both because E-H may generate misleading market definitions and because there is no necessary link between the number of sellers and market power under patient-driven competition. While there is a link between the number of sellers and market power under payer-driven competition, the link to patient travel is tenuous. An E-H analysis may overstate market size under payer-driven competition, for reasons that I outline in the next section.

A Simple Model of Pricing by a Local Monopolist

Suppose that at the time an individual requires hospitalization, he or she realizes a "value of access" that is random; that is, different individuals have different values. The patient may place a high value on local access if, for example, that patient has an ill family member, is suffering from a disability that limits travel, or otherwise has a strong

FIGURE 6–1
Profit under "Traditional" Pricing

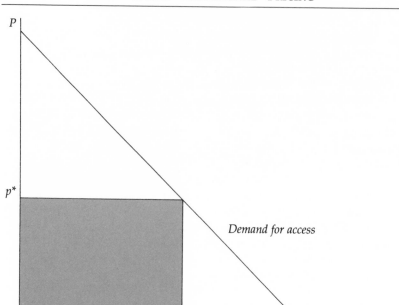

SOURCE: Author.

preference to remain close to home. I assume at first that all patients draw from the same distribution. This assumption is useful for demonstrating the different pricing problem facing providers under patient-driven and payer-driven competition.

Consider pricing under patient-driven competition of a hospital that is the only one in its locality. For simplicity, assume that costs are zero. Suppose that for any patient residing in that locality, the value of access ranges from $\underline{v}$ to $\bar{v}$, depending on circumstances at the time of illness. To exploit its local market power, the hospital considers raising its price by some amount p^*, where $\underline{v} \leq p^* \leq \bar{v}$. All patients who value local access by at least p^*, denoted $q^*(p)$, would continue to go to that hospital. By effectively charging for local access, the hospital would generate revenue of $p^* \leq q^*(p^*)$. This amount is the familiar monopoly profit rectangle, as depicted in figure 6–1.

If there were more than one hospital in the locality, they would compete for local patients. This might drive the access price toward zero. Of course, if they merged, they could charge for access without driving patients to a distant hospital.

Now suppose that patients select their hospital before realizing the value of local access. A hospital could charge an access fee to local patients. Patients who pay this fee in advance would be able to access the hospitals at the time they need care. Patients who refused to pay the fee would have to seek care elsewhere. In this example, the hospital could charge an amount equal to the expected value of access, which is the integral sum from $\underline{v}$ to $\bar{v}$. All patients would be willing to pay this amount, which equals the *total area under the access demand curve*, and therefore would exceed the monopoly profit rectangle discussed above. In this way the hospital could extract the total value of access from all patients and yet keep all its patients.

As before, competition between local hospitals may constrain their ability to profit from patient demand for local access. In this particular example, merging hospitals prosper more under payer-driven competition, as they capture a greater share of the value of local access (the entire area under the access demand curve instead of just the monopoly rectangle).

This result depends, in part, on the assumption that all patients place ex ante an identical value on local access. The model, however, may be generalized to the case where patients are not identical. Consider, for example, a group of employees with different demands for local access. Their employer wishes to select a provider network that will maximize the utility of its employees.[14] The local hospital could charge the employer an access fee equal to the average value of access across all employees, and the employer would still include it in the network. In this way, the hospital would extract the full value of access from every employee, just as in the previous model.

Hospitals do not, in reality, charge upfront access fees.[15] But they can raise the prices they charge to managed-care payers, with the same effect. Managed-care payers pass along these higher prices in the form of higher premiums, which have the same effect as upfront access fees in the sense that they are borne before the realization of illness. As before, competition among local hospitals may eliminate their ability to extract access fees.

---

14. It would be interesting to extend this analysis to other employer objective functions.

15. The reasons why they do not would be an interesting subject for research.

FIGURE 6–2
Convex Demand for Access

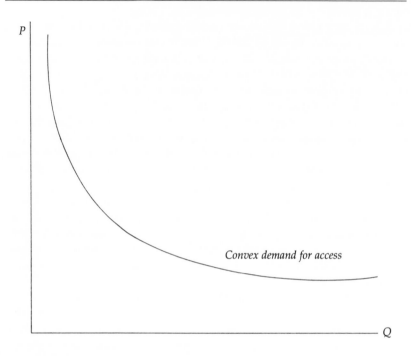

Convex demand for access

Source: Author.

These arguments show that local monopolists may be able to extract higher prices from patients who value local access, whether demand is patient driven or payer driven. The simple example presented above suggests that monopolists may do better under payer-driven competition. But this example is not entirely convincing. Suppose that patients place different values on local access. Then a hospital that charges an "upfront access fee" or the equivalent may drive some patients to select a plan that does not include it. Those patients would then visit another hospital, even if it turns out that they have a condition for which they highly value local access. For such patients at least, the hospital might have been better off setting a low upfront access fee. An interesting question is under what conditions a monopoly hospital prospers most by charging an access fee.

Some preliminary analyses suggest that if the demand for access is "convex," then a local monopoly hospital is better off charging an access fee. Figure 6–2 depicts convex demand for access. Convex demand is present if, for example, there is a substantial probability that the value of local access will be small, but on a few occasions that value will be very high. These high-value occasions drive up the average value of access in a way that is out of proportion to their probability of occurring. This increases the profit-maximizing price under payer-driven competition, when the hospital looks at the average value of access. But the profit-maximizing price under patient-driven competition is not necessarily changed, because the hospital must be concerned about driving away the bulk of its customers—customers who do not place a high value on access—by charging a high access fee. Hence, convex demand for access may enable a monopoly provider to earn greater profits under payer-driven competition.

We may speculate about other reasons why local monopoly providers may be more likely to exploit their market power under payer-driven competition. First, as discussed, pricing under patient-driven competition was very complex, with most studies failing to find a link between monopoly status and price. Most studies do find such a link under payer-driven competition. This evidence suggests that, for whatever reason, market power and pricing under payer-driven competition are more closely linked. Second, many hospitals, especially nonprofits, may have been reluctant to raise prices substantially merely to exploit patients who value local access highly. It is subtler, and more equitable, to charge a smaller access fee to all local residents than to charge a high fee at the time care is delivered. Third, managed care may facilitate price discrimination. In particular, providers may determine that different plans are contracting in behalf of different employers. Providers could then raise prices to those employers whose employees reside nearby. Last, providers may be willing to lose managed-care contracts if they believe that, as a result, employees who covet local access will instead select an indemnity policy. (Indemnity policies generally reimburse hospitals at higher rates.)

Implications of the Model for Market Definition. The model of access demand suggests that a firm may command a premium price if it faces little local competition, even if an E-H test shows that many local residents travel elsewhere for some medical care. While this result may hold for both patient- and payer-driven competition, there is some reason to suspect that it will be stronger under the payer driven. It seems appropriate, then, that antitrust analysis should augment data on patient flows with data on contracting.

To illustrate, consider the merger of two hospitals in Dubuque, Iowa, that was challenged by the Department of Justice (*U.S. v. Mercy Health Systems*, no. C94–1023). As in most recent mergers challenged by the Federal Trade Commission and the Department of Justice, the two hospitals appeared to many to be the largest in their market. (Mergers between smaller hospitals may conceivably be procompetitive, as they may create scale economies that force larger hospitals to lower prices.) In defending their merger, the two Dubuque hospitals sought to define as broad a geographic market as possible to make it appear that they faced many competitors. They commissioned a study in which some individuals indicated that they were willing to travel to another city to save an amount "less than $1,000." Combined with testimony from a managed-care purchaser that such inducements would cause at least some consumers to travel, the judge concluded that the geographic market was broad.

This was the wrong survey question, as it focused on access at the time of need. A better question would have focused on whether consumers would be willing to forgo all access during the year, regardless of circumstances. To determine the wording of a more appropriate question, consider that hospital costs typically account for about 40 percent of the total cost of a managed-care plan. Hence, if hospital prices were to go up by, say, $750, the managed-care plan cost would increase by around $300. The survey could have asked if individuals would purchase a managed-care plan that denied access to local hospitals but saved them $300. Better still, the survey could have asked local employers if they would be willing to offer, as their only managed-care plan, one that denied local access but saved $300.

The DOJ attempted to make this argument in the Dubuque case, but the judge believed that there was no difference between decision making by patients at the time of need and decision making by employers before need. But the model shows that this is not the case. As the model indicates, the local hospitals could charge higher prices without fear of losing contracts (and patients). It is quite possible that had a survey been administered with the "correct" question, the results would have indicated that the local hospitals could indeed have raised prices without losing contracts. The DOJ said that local hospitals did just that in a similar situation in Ottumwa, Iowa, but the judge ruled that opportunities for outside travel were sufficiently different in the two markets as to make the comparison irrelevant.

Although the discussion has focused largely on geographic market power, many of the concepts associated with the value of access also apply to other dimensions. Consumers may be reluctant to sign up for a managed-care plan that does not include a teaching hospital, a hospital with neonatology services, or the like. Convex preferences (that is, low probabilities of high need) work to enhance market power under payer-driven competition.

Conclusions

It is not clear whether traditional antitrust methods have ever been suited to antitrust inquiries into health care practices. Under patient-driven competition, the presumed connection between market structure and pricing was severed. Under payer-driven competition, traditional tools for both product and geographic market definition are wanting. At a time of unprecedented consolidation within the industry, it is essential that the appropriate tools be used in antitrust analysis. We have a number of reasons to believe that traditional methods may create a bias in favor of mergers that will turn out to harm consumers. If so, then a continued reliance on old methods and assumptions may lead to irreversible adverse consequences for health care consumers.

References

Allen, Henry, Grey Tucker, and David Dranove. 1989. "Antitrust Challenges to Hospital Mergers." *Health Lawyer* 3:1–10.

Barro, James, and David Cutler. 1997. "Consolidation in the Medical Care Marketplace: A Case Study from Massachusetts." NBER working paper no. 5957.

Bresnahan, Timothy. 1989. "Empirical Studies of Industries with Market Power." In R. Schmalensee and R. Willig, eds., *Handbook of Industrial Organization*. Amsterdam: North Holland.

Dranove, David, and William White. 1996. "Specialization, Option Demand, and the Pricing of Medical Specialists." *Journal of Economics and Management Strategy* 5:277–306.

Feldman, Roger, et al. 1990. "Effects of Health Maintenance Organizations on the Creation of Competitive Markets for Hospital Services." *Journal of Health Economics* 9:207–22.

Hogarty, Thomas, and Kenneth Elzinga. 1973. "The Problem of Geographic Market Delineation in Antimerger Suits." *Antitrust Bulletin* 28:45–81.

Werden, Greg. 1992. "Four Suggestions on Market Delineation." *Antitrust Bulletin* 37:107–21.

Who Profits from the Not-for-Profit Hospital? Proceedings of the George Bugbee Symposium. 1989. Conducted by the Graduate Program in Health Administration and Center for Health Administration Studies, University of Chicago.

7
Vertical Relations in Health Care Markets

Martin Gaynor and Deborah Haas-Wilson

The faces of health care markets as we know them are being changed dramatically. Managed care has been growing steadily as a percentage of the insurance market, and it now comprises 73 percent of all privately insured individuals (Jensen et al. 1997). One of the most salient aspects of managed care for the organization of health care markets is the increasing dominance of selective contracting for the provision of health care services. Managed-care organizations contract selectively with only a subset of providers in a market. This policy provides the managed-care organization with the bargaining power to extract lower prices from providers, and it can potentially provide the managed-care plan with greater control over utilization, cost, and quality. Selective contracting, in turn, sets into motion market forces that have led to a plethora of mergers, networks, joint ventures, and contracts between hospitals, physicians, and insurers.

While this dramatic change in the structure of health care markets has included extensive horizontal consolidation (Levin and Associates 1997), one of the unique aspects is the extent to which it is characterized by vertical associations (associations between firms operating in different, but related, product markets, such as insurers and hospitals, insurers and physicians, or physicians and hospitals). Physicians and hospitals are forming physician-hospital organizations (PHOs) and management service organizations (MSOs). Vertical integration and vertical contracts between insurers and providers are also increasing.

We wish to thank Jon Baker, David Dranove, Michael Morrisey, William Sage, William White, an anonymous referee, and participants in the AEI conference Managed Care and Changing Health Care Markets for helpful discussions and comments. Support was provided in part by a grant from the Robert Wood Johnson Foundation under the Investigators in Health Policy Research Program. The usual caveat applies.

These types of vertical relations between insurers and providers or hospitals and physicians are emerging as a key element of competition in health care markets. The number of physician practices owned or managed by hospital-based systems increased by 60 percent between 1994 and 1995, from 7,015 to 11,234 (*Modern Healthcare* 1996). Columbia/HCA, the largest for-profit hospital chain, attempted to acquire Blue Cross/Blue Shield of Ohio, but state regulators disapproved the merger in March 1997. Allina, an HMO in Minneapolis, has been acquiring hospitals and physician practices. Blue Cross of Western Pennsylvania has been purchasing physician practices. Kaiser Permanente Health Plan in Dallas signed an exclusive, five-year contract with Columbia/HCA in January 1995 (*Managed Care Week* 1995). Further, providers are integrating into the market for insurance by starting to bear insurance risk. For example, Promina Health Systems in Atlanta, Georgia, applied for an HMO license in 1996, because Georgia requires licensure of providers that take capitation from self-insured employers (*Managed Care Week* 1996).

There is also some evidence of a trend toward looser vertical associations (a trend away from vertical integration and exclusive contracts) between insurers and providers. In March 1997, Aetna U.S. Healthcare sold its physician practices to Medpartners, the largest physician management company, and signed a ten-year, nonexclusive contract with Medpartners to provide services to Aetna U.S. Healthcare's HMO enrollees (*Modern Healthcare* 1997). In 1996, FHP International Corp., an HMO, announced plans to spin off its physician practice management company in order to allow the physicians to better compete for business from other insurers. Foundation Health Corp., PacifiCare Health Systems, and Physician Corp. of America are other HMOs that sold their physician operations in 1996 (*Modern Healthcare* 1996).

The implications of this reorganization for health care competition, and thus for costs, quality, and innovation, are profound. The key question is, To what extent will these new vertical associations in health care markets enhance efficiency and quality, and to what extent will they facilitate collusion, monopoly power, and higher prices or lower quality?

We argue that the blessing of managed care is that it can do a lot to solve the agency problems between hospitals and physicians or insurer and health care providers. The classic problem between insurers and providers (or between hospitals and physicians) is that providers' decisions affect the insurers' costs and quality, and consequently their competitive positions or profits, but insurers have not had effective mechanisms for aligning providers' incentives with their own or with directly controlling providers' decisions. As we indicate in what follows, the promise or blessing of managed care is the potential to offer substantial progress toward internalizing this vertical externality. The curse of managed care is the increasing potential for anticompetitive behavior, especially vertical foreclosure and horizontal collusion. As firms have consolidated across product markets, concerns about such vertical arrangements foreclosing competitors from the market, reducing competition, and increasing the potential to exercise monopoly power have emerged.

Economists are still debating the competitive effects of vertical associations, and so far there is little agreement. The Chicago School concludes that vertical integration and vertical restraints do not have anticompetitive effects, while the post–Chicago School argues that vertical integration and vertical restraints can be anticompetitive under certain conditions. We discuss the differences between the models used by the two schools in an attempt to explain why reasonable people can come to such different conclusions. We also address the issue of which model best describes competition in health care markets.

Given this continuing debate and the newness of the proliferation of vertical integration and restraints in health care markets, it is not surprising that there are many unsettled antitrust policy issues concerning vertical associations in health care markets. For example, the Department of Justice (DOJ) and Federal Trade Commission (FTC) Statements of Antitrust Enforcement Policy in Health Care (August 1996) lay out "antitrust safety zones" for horizontal provider arrangements, such as hospital mergers or joint ventures and physician network joint ventures, but not for vertical provider arrangements. These safety zones describe a subset of the types of provider arrangements that the agencies are unlikely to challenge under the antitrust laws. The agencies were not able to lay out safety zones for vertical provider arrangements. "Because multiprovider networks involve a large variety of structures and relationships among many different types of health care providers, and new arrangements are continually developing, the agencies are unable to establish a meaningful safety zone for these entities" (DOJ/FTC, 80–81).

The legal status of most-favored-nation (MFN) clauses is another example of an unsettled antitrust issue involving vertical restraints in health care markets. The legal status of MFN contract clauses under the antitrust laws is still evolving. Recent court decisions have upheld MFN clauses on the presumption that MFN clauses are not anticompetitive. Judge Posner in the Marshfield Clinic case characterized MFN clauses as "the sort of conduct that the antitrust laws seek to encourage."[1] Between 1994 and 1996, however, the DOJ and the FTC have

---

1. Blue Cross and Blue Shield v. Marshfield Clinic, 65 F.3d 1406, 1415 (7th Cir. 1995) at 1415.

challenged the MFN clauses in three statewide dental insurance plans (Delta Dental Plan of Arizona, Oregon Dental Services, and Delta Dental of Rhode Island), a national vision care insurer (Vision Service Plan), and a statewide pharmacy network (RxCare of Tennessee) as unreasonable vertical restraints.

The potential procompetitive and anticompetitive effects of vertical integration and vertical restraints are the focus of this chapter. We explore the implications of the new vertical restraints emerging in health care markets for efficiency enhancement and competition. The following section discusses managed care and vertical associations, the next section reviews economic thinking on vertical associations, and the ensuing three sections analyze the potential effects of vertical integration, exclusive dealing agreements, and MFN clauses, respectively, in health care markets and recent health care antitrust cases. Antitrust has emerged as a crucial element of health policy. The potential for market forces to constrain health care costs is, in part, determined by the enforcement of the antitrust laws that are designed to ensure that competition will lead to competitive rather than anticompetitive behavior. The final section contains a summary and conclusions.

Managed Care and Vertical Associations

Perhaps the most distinctive aspect of current changes in the structure of health care markets is the growth of vertical associations.[2] As insurers, physicians, and hospitals form integrated delivery systems, merge, sign exclusive contracts, and form alliances, the lines between the traditional markets have blurred. Rather than consumers choosing the firms from which they want to buy in each market (in essence, acting as their own general contractor for their health care), they are now offered packages of insurance and health services. Managed-care organizations (MCOs) act as selective contractors of services from providers. Managed-care selective contracting often involves exclusion of certain providers, since typically MCOs sign contracts for service provision with only a subset of the available providers in a market. Further, selective contracting encourages the formation of provider networks, such as physician networks, and multiprovider networks,

---

2. In this chapter we concentrate on vertical restraints. Consequently, while monopsony is a vertical association, we do not cover the exercise of monopsony power in this chapter. We also do not discuss tying. While this is a vertical restraint, it has not yet arisen as a prominent issue associated with managed care.

such as physician-hospital organizations (PHOs), that often involve exclusion of certain providers.

Selective contracting by MCOs and the growth of multiprovider networks give rise to a variety of vertical associations, ranging from vertical integration to nonexclusive contracts. The most controversial vertical associations found in health care markets include vertical integration, vertical joint ventures, exclusive contracts, and most-favored-nation (MFN) clauses.[3] Vertical integration represents one end of the spectrum in that it involves two firms becoming one; for example, a staff-model HMO. Exclusive contracts or exclusive dealing agreements involve agreements on the part of at least one of the parties in the exchange to trade only with the other. Vertical joint ventures are collaborative associations involving partial integration among providers and insurers or hospitals and physicians. For example, a hospital and an insurer may form a joint venture to offer a new HMO. MFN clauses are vertical contractual agreements in which the seller (for example, a hospital or physician group/network) agrees not to charge the buyer (for example, an insurer) more than the lowest price it charges any other buyer. If the seller offers another buyer a lower price, then the seller must offer the same lower price to the buyer with the MFN clause.

Economic Thinking on Vertical Associations

One line of investigation in the economics literature has been concerned with understanding the potential efficiencies associated with vertical integration and vertical restraints, such as exclusive dealing agreements.

Efficiency Gains from Vertical Associations. Both vertical integration and vertical restraints can be efficiency enhancing by leading to more efficient input pricing, lowering transaction costs, ensuring supply of an input, improving coordination between the firms, and improving monitoring (Williamson 1989; Carlton and Perloff 1994; Riordan and Salop 1995). This literature refers to upstream and downstream firms. Downstream firms are potential customers of the upstream firms. Accordingly, in vertical associations between retailers and manufacturers, the retailers would be the downstream firms and manufacturers would be the upstream firms. In vertical relations between input suppliers and manufacturers, however, the manufacturers would be the down-

---

3. These are also referred to as "most-favored-customer" clauses. The terms are used interchangeably.

stream firms. In health care markets, health care providers would be upstream firms, and insurers would be downstream firms.

If the upstream firm in a vertical relation possesses market power, vertical relations (specifically exclusive dealing or integration) can increase efficiency by leading to more efficient input pricing. The problem occurs if there is a monopoly in the input market combined with a monopoly in the output market, or if the firm in the output market is both a monopsony and a monopoly.[4] In both these cases the input is not priced at marginal cost, leading to inefficient use of the input and inefficient levels of the output. This is well known as the "double marginalization" or "successive monopoly" result (Spengler 1950). For example, if a monopoly hospital is selling to a monopoly insurer, the hospital sells to the insurer at a price set above its marginal cost, and the insurer marks up the price again. In an integrated firm or with exclusive dealing, the hospital will "sell" its inputs to the insurer at marginal cost, thus eliminating the double markup and increasing output and thereby social welfare.

Merger or tight contractual arrangements between upstream and downstream firms may also increase efficiency by lowering the costs of their transactions. Transaction costs include the costs of negotiating, writing, monitoring, and enforcing contracts. Transaction costs are especially high when there is uncertainty, and thus it is costly to negotiate contracts with all possible contingencies; when there are few alternative suppliers, and hence opportunities for opportunistic behavior; or when extensive coordination among the firms at the different stages of production is required (Coase 1937; Williamson 1975). All three of these conditions are present in markets for health care. An insurer that is integrated with a set of physicians or who deals contractually with the same set of physicians on a repeated basis may have significantly lower transaction costs than one who deals with a changing group of physician suppliers. Similarly, physicians may have significantly lower costs by transacting with a single insurer, as opposed to writing and maintaining contracts with multiple insurers on an individual basis.[5]

---

4. Inefficiency can result simply from monopoly in the input market. Without monopoly power in the output market, however, there is no incentive for the monopoly firm in the input market to integrate with a firm in the output market.

5. It has been argued that one of the foremost reasons for the observed higher administrative costs of health care in the United States in comparison with other countries is the costs that insurers and providers bear by transacting with a large and changing set of partners.

145

Vertical merger or exclusive dealing may also help in ensuring supply of an input. Insurers offering managed-care plans offer a network of providers as part of a plan. Ensuring that there is a sufficient supply of providers of all sorts is important. In particular, ensuring supply of a scarce or critical input is particularly important. In health care this takes the form of a specialized service; thus, it is critical for managed-care plans to ensure the supply of services from specialized physicians or hospital facilities (see Dranove and White 1997 for more on this point). If buyers of managed-care plans want to be assured access to a hospital with organ transplant services, it will be important to managed-care plans to ensure the supply of services from this hospital. Assurance of access to a specialized service can come about through vertical integration, exclusive dealing, or long-term contracting.[6]

Monitoring and controlling quantity or quality may be done more efficiently in organizations where upstream and downstream firms are vertically integrated or have long-term contracts, and thus share similar goals and aligned incentives. Independent firms may work at cross purposes. A classic problem in health care is the external effects or spillovers of providers' decisions on insurers.[7] For example, when an independent physician decides to provide lower quality care to a patient, the physician will consider the costs of lowering quality to his or her own reputation, demand, and income, but may not consider the costs of lowering quality to the hospital's or insurer's reputation, demand, and profits. Vertical integration or close contractual relations provide the opportunity to align incentives across firms, and in this example the opportunity to increase quality. Similarly, insurers' incentives to make investments or engage in expenditures on behalf of providers (for example, promotional activities) are considerably strengthened by integration or exclusive dealing.

Further, to the extent that monitoring activities are specific to the relationship between an upstream and a downstream firm (for example, a provider and an insurer) and necessitate fixed investments, it may be very costly for an upstream firm to do monitoring to the differing specifications of multiple downstream firms. Dealing with a single downstream firm may provide the economies necessary for an up-

---

6. See Dranove and White (1996, 1997) on how this can confer market power on such a facility.

7. Research in health economics has concentrated on the efficiency effects of vertical relations between insurers and providers, specifically on the design of incentive contracts to control consumer and provider agency problems (see Gaynor 1994 for a survey).

stream firm to invest in monitoring systems. In health care, this often occurs as investments by providers in information systems and review protocols for the monitoring of utilization, costs, and quality of care, subject to the specifications of insurers. Another point is that such investments are more likely to take place in the context of a long-term continuing relationship, where the provider has more assurance of recouping a return on its investment. Integration or close contractual ties constitute such a relationship.

Anticompetitive Concerns about Vertical Relations. The economics literature on vertical restraints derived originally as a response to early antitrust case law in this area. Early court decisions were extremely restrictive in their treatment of vertical integration or exclusionary practices.[8] The courts expressed concern that vertical integration or exclusive deals could lead to market foreclosure and consequently be harmful to competition. The intent was clearly to keep markets unconcentrated by stopping any trend toward concentration in its incipiency.[9]

Strong criticism of case law by the Chicago School led to a new perspective in which exclusive dealing (and other forms of vertical relations) were viewed as competitively neutral or procompetitive (Bork 1978). This view underpins the liberal 1985 Department of Justice Vertical Restraints Guidelines and the permissive policy toward vertical restraints exercised during the Reagan and Bush administrations. Currently, concern about vertical restraints has been renewed. One of former Assistant Attorney General Bingaman's first official acts was to repeal the 1985 Vertical Restraints Guidelines. The Department of Justice and the Federal Trade Commission have initiated actions against vertical restraints (see Riordan and Salop 1995).

---

8. For example, U.S. v. Aluminum Co. of America, 148 F.2d 416 (2nd Cir. 1945); Lorain Journal v. U.S., 342 U.S. 143 (1951), United Shoe Machinery Corp. v. U.S., 258 U.S. 451, 458 (1922) for exclusionary practices and Brown Shoe Co., Inc. v. U.S., 370 U.S. 294 (1962); A.G. Spalding & Bros., Inc., 56 F.T.C. 1125 (1960); Kennecott Copper Corp. v. U.S. 381 U.S. 414 (1965); Ford Motor Co. v. U.S. 381 U.S. 414 (1965); Ford Motor Co. v. U.S., 405 U.S. 562 (1972) for vertical integration.

9. In the Brown Shoe case, since Brown, primarily a shoe manufacturer, integrated forward with Kinney, primarily a retailer, the size of the market foreclosed to other manufacturers was 1.6 percent of the national market, Kinney's market share. Similarly, in the Ford Motor Co. (1972) case, the court held that Ford's acquisition of Autolite, a spark plug manufacturer, foreclosed other spark plug manufacturers, when Ford was a purchaser of only 10 percent of the total spark plug industry output.

The policy interest in vertical restraints is mirrored in the economics literature as well. Most recently, a post–Chicago School approach to vertical relations has emerged. Current thinking on vertical relations builds on the Chicago School critique by applying modern industrial organization theory to the analysis of more realistic market structures and conduct. This literature identifies situations in which exclusive dealing and other vertical restraints can raise concerns about competition.[10] In what follows, we review the Chicago School and the post–Chicago thinking on vertical restraints.

To illustrate the basic thinking behind foreclosure theories, consider relations between firms in upstream and downstream markets. We consider backward integration here by the downstream firm into the upstream market, but the intuition holds for forward integration as well. First consider a monopolist in the upstream market. If a downstream firm integrates or signs an exclusive deal with the upstream monopoly, it appears as if the other downstream firms are foreclosed from the market. Now consider an industry structure with multiple firms in both the upstream and downstream markets. If an upstream firm merges or signs an exclusive deal with a downstream firm, the remaining upstream firms face less competition and thus may be able to raise their prices. The downstream rivals of the integrated firm face higher costs and thus are at a competitive disadvantage.

The Chicago School critique of antitrust policy toward vertical integration and exclusive dealing consists of three main points. First, vertical integration or exclusive dealing between a downstream firm and an upstream supplier does not necessarily imply that the net supply of inputs to rival downstream firms is reduced.[11] In the example above with multiple upstream firms, rival downstream firms may now have access to other suppliers previously utilized by the firm involved in the merger or the exclusive deal. Just because access to one supplier is foreclosed does not mean that the net supply of inputs has been foreclosed. In addition, entry can occur in the upstream market, either by independent entrants or by the excluded downstream firms themselves. So even if there is an upstream monopoly, vertical integration or exclusive dealing does not necessarily imply foreclosure. Second, the Chicago School claims that a monopolist cannot enhance its mo-

---

10. This literature has been criticized in turn for demonstrating only the possible existence of anticompetitive effects and not considering efficiency enhancing impacts (see Klass and Salinger 1995).

11. This applies similarly to the consideration of upstream firms' access to a buyer if an upstream firm merges or engages in an exclusive deal with a downstream firm.

nopoly power by the use of exclusive dealing or other vertical restraints. There is a "single monopoly profit," regardless of the nature of vertical relations (Bork 1978, 229). In the case of the upstream monopolist above, the upstream firm has nothing to gain from such a merger, since it is already maximizing its profits by selling to the entire downstream industry as a monopolist. This intuition also applies to market power generally. Bork states,

> Vertical merger does not create or increase the firm's power to restrict output. The ability to restrict output depends on the share of the market occupied by the firm. Horizontal mergers increase market share, but vertical mergers do not. [1978, 231]

Third, the Chicago School criticizes the case law on forward integration on the grounds that upstream firms could not induce downstream firms to accept exclusionary contracts if such contracts actually hurt the downstream firms (Director and Levi 1956). This applies to backward integration as well. In the case with multiple upstream firms above, if the unintegrated upstream firms gain market power as a result of the vertical merger, the upstream firm approached by the downstream firm has an incentive to remain unintegrated. The downstream firm must compensate an upstream partner for lost profits, potentially rendering the deal unprofitable. Posner (1976, 212) and Bork (1978, 309) conclude that exclusionary contracts cannot cause any harm and therefore ought to be disregarded by antitrust law. The Chicago School conclusion is that since there are no anticompetitive effects of vertical integration or exclusive dealing, these vertical restraints will exist only where they result in efficiencies, hence they must be beneficial.

The Chicago School view is based on economic models that employ strong assumptions. In particular, the result of a single monopoly profit depends critically on the assumptions of a fixed proportions technology, perfect competition in the upstream or input market, and monopoly in the downstream or output market with prohibitive barriers to entry.[12] The results are critically sensitive to these assumptions (Riordan and Salop 1995; Westfield 1981; Vernon and Graham 1971). These assumptions do not hold in most markets and certainly do not hold in health care markets.

Proponents of the post–Chicago School argue that vertical restraints can enhance efficiency, but also that vertical restraints can be anticompetitive under certain conditions. The anticompetitive effects

---

12. Note that the single monopoly profit result and its criticisms apply as well to the case of forward integration, in which there is a monopoly in the input market and perfect competition in the output market.

of vertical restraints come from: (1) the potential for a vertically related firm to raise rivals' costs or foreclose rivals' access to a necessary market and (2) the potential for vertical relations to confer market power by facilitating horizontal coordination or collusion. The argument for foreclosure, as indicated previously, has suffered from some weaknesses. The post–Chicago School has attempted to use modern game theory to construct theories that are internally consistent and address these weaknesses (Ordover, Saloner, and Salop 1990; Salinger 1988; Hart and Tirole 1990; Riordan 1996; Choi and Yi 1996). We provide more detail on these theories in the next section.

In health care markets, vertical relations between hospitals (or physician groups and networks) and insurers may raise the costs of rival insurers, raise the costs of potential entrants into the insurance market, or increase the ability of insurers to collude and thus increase the ability of the insurer with the vertical relation to increase prices or lower quality. For example, if there are multiple insurers in a market but only one hospital, then a merger or an exclusive contract between one of the insurers and the hospital has the potential to be anticompetitive. The vertically related insurer and hospital may choose not to sell hospital services to the other insurance firms, thereby completely foreclosing the other insurers' access to the hospital services market and rendering them unable to compete. Or the vertically related insurer and hospital may sell hospital services to the rival insurers, but at a price higher than the internal cost to the vertically related firm. This puts the rival insurers at a competitive disadvantage, forcing them to sell at higher prices, thus allowing the vertically related firm to sell insurance at a price above its cost, but still remain competitive.[13]

Alternatively, vertical integration, exclusive contracts, or other forms of vertical restraints between an upstream firm and a downstream firm may foreclose other upstream firms' access to downstream markets. This may raise the costs of rival firms in the upstream market, thus bestowing market power on the firm with the vertical restraint. In health care markets, vertical relations between hospitals and physicians may raise the costs of rival hospitals and raise the costs of potential entrants into the hospital market, thus increasing the ability of the vertically related hospital to exercise market power by raising price or lowering quality. For example, if there are multiple hospitals but only one major physician group, then a merger or an exclusive contract be-

---

13. An alternate example of two hospitals and one insurer would work exactly the same way, with vertical integration or exclusive dealing foreclosing one of the hospitals and bestowing market power in the hospital market on the merged firm.

tween one of the hospitals and the physician group has the potential to be anticompetitive. The vertically related physician group may not admit patients to the other hospitals, thereby completely foreclosing the other hospitals and rendering them unable to compete. Or the vertically related physician group may admit patients to rival hospitals but admit only the least profitable patients to rival hospitals. This would put rival hospitals at a competitive disadvantage, forcing them to sell at higher prices, thus allowing the vertically related firm to sell hospital services at a price above its costs but still remain competitive.

Another concern with vertical restraints is that they may act as facilitating devices, leading to horizontal collusion. For example, if a downstream firm is integrated with an upstream input supplier but continues to buy inputs from other upstream firms, then it will receive price quotes and other information from these firms. It can also transmit information from the integrated upstream firm to the other upstream firms. This information can be used to facilitate collusive practices in the upstream market (Riordan and Salop 1995). In addition, an increase in the market power of a firm through a vertical agreement may provide it with sufficient power to initiate or enforce collusive horizontal behavior.

The antitrust policy implications of this post–Chicago School view are that vertical relations should be judged under the rule of reason: in other words the benefits, or efficiencies, associated with the vertical relations should be weighed against the costs, or anticompetitive effects.

Vertical Integration

Despite the prevalence of vertical integration in real-world industries, the theoretical literature on its competitive effects is relatively small and recent. The literature on the competitive effects of vertical integration includes papers by Salinger (1988), Ordover, Saloner, and Salop (1990), Hart and Tirole (1990), Bolton and Whinston (1993), Riordan (1996), and Choi and Yi (1996). These papers demonstrate that vertical integration sometimes can lead to monopolization outcomes, concluding that vertical integration may be anticompetitive. In the literature, a key issue concerns the incentive of a vertically integrated firm to sell intermediate inputs to other downstream firms. The foreclosure effect obtains only if a vertically integrated firm refuses to sell intermediate inputs, or sells at a higher price, so that nonintegrated downstream firms must pay a higher input price and compete at a disadvantage against the integrated firm. Whether such a foreclosure incentive can

result as an equilibrium in a rigorous model has been the main research question in these papers.[14]

Riordan's (1996) model of vertical integration by a dominant upstream firm illustrates a circumstance in which vertical merger can be
anticompetitive. For example, consider an insurance market with a
dominant firm and a competitive fringe, and a competitive physician-
services market with rising marginal costs.[15] The dominant firm has
monopoly power in the insurance market and monopsony power in
the physician-services market. If the dominant insurer integrates backward into the physician-services market it will no longer act like a mo-
nopsonist in that market, and hence will purchase more physician
services. This will increase the price of physician services to the fringe
insurers, because of upward sloping supply. This reduces the size of
the fringe and deters entry in the insurance market, thus increasing the
power of the dominant firm in this market and allowing it to increase
its price.[16] Exclusive dealing could have the same effect.

Ordover, Saloner, and Salop (1990) do not rely on a dominant
firm. They examine a market with two upstream and two downstream
firms. They show that if the vertically integrated firm can commit to
selling its input to the unintegrated downstream firm at a price above
marginal cost then integration can lead to a foreclosure effect by raising the costs of the downstream rival. The problem with this result,
however, is that the integrated firm has a strong incentive to sell at a
price below that to which it has committed in order to undercut the
independent upstream firm. This leads to its pricing at marginal cost,
and thus there is no foreclosure (Reiffen 1992). Choi and Yi (1996) establish foreclosure in a similar model by allowing cost-reducing investments as a means of commitment. The integrated firm has an incentive
to engage in the investments and thus can credibly commit itself to the
higher input price, establishing a foreclosure equilibrium. While these
papers consider backward integration and foreclosure in the downstream market, the issues are essentially the same for forward integration and upstream foreclosure.

---

14. The results can be somewhat fragile. For example, the results of Ordover, Saloner, and Salop (1990) depend critically on an assumption that the
integrated firm can commit to sell to the unintegrated downstream firm at a
higher price than the internal transfer price within the integrated firm (Reiffen
1992). Some more recent papers are less sensitive to assumptions (Riordan
1996; Choi and Yi 1996).

15. One of the authors resides in an area in which these markets might be
characterized in precisely this way.

16. This is the result of theorem 1 in Riordan (1996), presented in a health
care setting.

Two recent health care antitrust cases illustrate some of the issues related to vertical integration and the potential for foreclosure in health care markets. First, these cases illustrate that charges of foreclosure occur in both upstream and downstream markets. In the *Vicksburg Clinic* case, the plaintiff charged that hospital-physician integration would foreclose a nonintegrated hospital from the upstream market for hospital services. In the *Marshfield Clinic* case, the plaintiff charged that physician-HMO integration had foreclosed a nonintegrated HMO from the downstream market for health care financing. Second, these cases illustrate that vertical integration will be found to have anticompetitive effects only where the vertically integrated firm has market power in the upstream or downstream market. Market power, in turn, depends on the presence of barriers to entry. In both these cases the courts ruled that vertical integration did not or would not lead to foreclosure, because the vertically integrated firms lacked market power.

The antitrust case in Vicksburg, Mississippi, concerned the proposed merger between Vicksburg Clinic, one of the two largest physician groups in town, and River Regional, a physician-owned integrated delivery system that included the other large physician group and one of Vicksburg's two hospitals. Columbia Vicksburg Medical Center, the other hospital in town, challenged the merger on both horizontal and vertical grounds. First, Columbia charged that the merger would lessen competition in the markets for physician services and hospital services, and in the managed-care market. Second, Columbia charged that the merger would foreclose Columbia from the hospital-services market by giving the physicians of the Vicksburg Clinic the financial incentive to shift their patient admissions to the hospital associated with River Regional.[17] In other words, Columbia charged that if the merger were allowed, then the vertically integrated River Regional would have the ability to foreclose the nonintegrated upstream firm (Columbia) from the market for hospital services by refusing to buy inputs (hospital services) or buying fewer inputs from Columbia.

For Columbia to prevail on its vertical claim, it had to prove that the merging firms would have market power in the physician-services market. This could be true if entry into the physician-services market in Vicksburg were difficult. In particular, if managed care is important, and if managed care prefers to contract with a network of physicians rather than with individual practices, the sunk costs of entering as a network could constitute a barrier to entry. On March 4, 1997, however, the court ruled that despite River Region's high postmerger market

---

17. The physicians would become postmerger equity shareholders in River Regional.

share in the market for primary care physician services (calculated as 58 or 70 percent), Columbia had not established that the merged firm would have market power, because there are low barriers to entry into the market for primary care physician services.[18] Further, the court ruled that there was no credible evidence that financial incentives would cause the Vicksburg Clinic physicians to shift hospital patient admissions to the hospital associated with River Regional and that there was evidence that patients, rather than physicians, select the hospital.

In the other recent health care case, Blue Cross/Blue Shield (BC/BS) of Wisconsin charged that Marshfield Clinic, a physician-owned clinic that is vertically integrated with its HMO, had excluded the BC/BS HMO from the health care–financing market by monopolizing the market for physician services. On appeal, however, the court ruled that the facts of the case did not support these charges.[19] The court found that Marshfield Clinic did not have market power in the market for physician services, and thus could not foreclose the BC/BS HMO from the market for health care financing.[20]

Marshfield Clinic employed about 400 physicians and contracted with approximately 900 additional physicians through its HMO, a very large share of physicians in the market. These physician contracts were not exclusive, however. Although the BC/BS HMO and the physician employees of the Marshfield Clinic were unable to agree on contract terms (and thus physician employees of Marshfield were not supplying services to the BC/BS HMO), the contracting physicians were not restrained from contracting to provide services for other HMOs and could practice fee-for-service medicine. Thus, the judge ruled that the vertical integration of the 400-physician Marshfield Clinic and its HMO could not have foreclosed the BC/BS HMO from the market for health care financing.

Exclusive Dealing Agreements or Exclusive Contracts

The effect of exclusive dealing agreements depends critically on the nature of the contract. The key factors are the degree of exclusivity of

---

18. HTI Health Services, Inc. vs. Quorum Health Group, Inc., River Regional Medical Corporation, and Vicksburg Clinic, P.A. U.S. District Court for the Southern District of Mississippi, Western Division (Civil Action No. 5:96-CV-108Br(S)).

19. Blue Cross/Blue Shield United of Wisconsin and Compcare Health Services Insurance Corporation v. Marshfield Clinic and Security Health Plan of Wisconsin in the U.S. Court of Appeals for the Seventh Circuit (Nos. 95–1965, 95–2140).

20. The ruling on this case is controversial. For an examination of a number of the other issues in the case see Sage (1997).

the contract, the length of the contract, and the penalties for breach of the contract. The degree of exclusivity is the extent to which one party is required either to sell or to buy services only from the other party. A provider's contract with a managed-care organization that has no exclusivity in it will have less effect than one that requires the provider to provide services only to the managed-care organization's enrollees. The length of contract is simply the length of the time period covered by the contract. For example, if that period is very short, say thirty days, one would not expect such a contract to have much effect, either for good or for bad. Last, the penalty for breach of contract will determine the force of that contract. Even if a contract is totally exclusive and very long term, if the penalty for abrogating that contract is trivial, the contract would not be expected to have much of an effect.

The major objection to exclusive dealing agreements is that they can lead to market foreclosure and facilitating horizontal collusion, thereby damaging competition and reducing social welfare. The issues here are the same as those concerning vertical integration. Thus, whether there is foreclosure critically depends on whether an exclusive deal reduces the net supply of inputs to rival firms in the downstream market. If access is reduced, then exclusive dealing agreements will raise the cost of doing business to rival firms (Krattenmaker and Salop 1986a, 1986b; Salop and Scheffman 1983, 1987). This will put rival downstream firms at a cost disadvantage, increase the market power and the profits of the downstream firm with the exclusive deal, and reduce social welfare (Katz 1989; Comanor and Frech 1985; Mathewson and Winter 1987; Schwartz 1987).[21] Not only can this deter entry into the downstream market or increase the unilateral market power of the downstream firm with exclusive contracts, it can make collusive agreements among downstream firms more likely. An increase in the market power of the firm with exclusive contracts can provide it with the necessary power to implement and enforce collusive agreements (Riordan and Salop 1995).

The crucial criticism to this line of reasoning is why an upstream firm (or downstream firm in the case of forward exclusive dealing) would sign an exclusive contract. As indicated previously, the Chicago School's position is that exclusive deals could not be anticompetitive,

---

21. Comanor and Frech claim to show that an exclusive deal can be anticompetitive by raising rivals' costs of entry. Mathewson and Winter and Schwartz are comments on the generality and technical validity of Comanor and Frech's results. Mathewson and Winter show that the relevant focus is on potential competition, not only actual competition. Schwartz shows that Comanor and Frech, by ignoring downstream firms' responses, have not constructed a subgame perfect equilibrium.

because if they were they would leave upstream firms worse off and rational firms would not sign a contract that reduces their welfare. Recent theoretical work shows, however, that it is possible to find an exclusionary equilibrium if it is not possible for the upstream firms to coordinate with each other (Aghion and Bolton 1987; Katz 1989; Rasmusen et al. 1991).

The health economics literature on exclusive contracts is scant. Three recent papers consider the effects of exclusive dealing between insurers and providers on competition in the insurance market. Gaynor and Ma (1996) consider differentiated health care providers and homogeneous insurers. Thus providers possess some market power, but the insurance market is perfectly competitive. Individuals, however, do not know which provider they will prefer should they fall ill, and they are risk neutral with regard to this uncertainty, so in essence health care providers are homogeneous ex ante. Since exclusive dealing means that both the insurer and the provider must be chosen ex ante, this effectively eliminates the differentiation between the providers. There is no anticompetitive effect in equilibrium, since the insurance market is perfectly competitive. Further, there is no ability to commit. The result is that exclusive dealing cannot create market power where there was none. Gal-Or (1996) considers the same problem, but with differentiated insurers. With differentiated insurers foreclosure can occur in equilibrium. In this case, a provider who agrees to an exclusive deal with an insurer will likely accept a lower payment rate in return for a larger volume of patients. If both insurers sign exclusive deals with different providers, this benefits insurers by reducing the outside options of the providers and thus reducing their payment rates. Encinosa (1996) considers exclusive deals between HMOs and physician groups. There is an incumbent HMO that has a cost advantage over a rival, but must invest in order to serve the entire market. When the incumbent HMO is risk averse, it may engage in an exclusive deal with the single provider. This will result in foreclosure and is socially inefficient.

Most-Favored-Nation Contract Clauses

Most-favored-nation clauses, also called most-favored-customer clauses, are vertical contractual agreements in which the seller (for example, a hospital or physician group or network) agrees not to charge the buyer (for example, an insurer) more than the lowest price it charges any other buyer. If the seller offers another buyer a lower price, then the seller must offer the same lower price to the buyer with the MFN clause. MFN clauses have appeared in contracts between health care providers and HMOs, Blue Cross/Blue Shield plans, managed dental plans, pharmacy networks (RxCare of Tennessee), and vision care insurers.

Recent work on MFN contracts also shows that such contracts can have anticompetitive effects in some situations; however, Chicago School analysts have interpreted MFN clauses as simply representing efforts by firms to obtain low prices and therefore as promoting competition (Posner 1995). Indeed, the fact that firms are willing to sign such contracts is interpreted as evidence that such contracts must not be harmful.

Modern theoretical analyses find, however, both that MFN clauses have the potential to be anticompetitive (Salop 1986; Cooper 1986; Baker 1996) and efficiency enhancing (P'ng 1991; Cooper and Fries 1995).[22] The main potential procompetitive effect is that MFN clauses may allow insurers or other buyers of health care services to lower their costs, and therefore to increase output or lower insurance prices. Baker (1996) argues that MFN clauses will most likely allow insurers to purchase health care services at lower prices in markets with many other insurers and in markets where it is costly for insurers to shop for lower prices. If one insurer can negotiate lower fees from health care providers, then the insurer with the MFN clause can ride free on that insurer's negotiating efforts and pay the lower fees without having to price shop or negotiate. Baker (1996) suggests, however, that competition among insurers may lead to a proliferation of contracts with MFN clauses, and this proliferation of MFN clauses increases providers' costs of discounting. In this case, providers may not offer discounts to insurers, and the efficiency justification for MFN clauses disappears. In other words, insurers may not be able to purchase inputs for less.

MFN clauses may impair horizontal competition in at least two ways. First, MFN clauses may facilitate tacit coordination (Salop 1986). Cooper (1986) shows in a two-period differentiated product duopoly model that both firms earn higher profits if at least one firm offers an MFN clause. MFN clauses may decrease competition among health care providers by reducing providers' incentives to offer lower prices to insurers. Since any discount the provider grants to another insurer means granting the discount to its partner in the MFN contract, the provider must grant the discount on all the inframarginal units it sells to its partner. This makes price reductions very costly and may be a way to signal a commitment to collusive pricing. Further, MFN clauses may reduce insurers' incentives to bargain with providers for lower

---

22. Corts (1996), however, finds that MFN clauses can be competitive and welfare enhancing.

prices, since rival insurers with MFN clauses would reap the benefits of the lower prices too. If MFN clauses facilitate coordination among providers and discourage selective discounting, then MFN clauses will lead to higher prices for health care services or lower quality health care services. The limiting factor on this behavior is the ease of entry or expansion into the market. If potential competitors or existing rivals can enter or expand easily, then the anticompetitive effects of MFN contracts will be limited. As mentioned in the previous discussion of the Vicksburg case, it is possible that the propensity of managed-care plans to contract with networks of providers acts as a barrier to entry into that market. If that is the case, then the success of MFN contracts in discouraging competition may be more likely in markets with more managed care.

Second, MFN clauses may increase rival insurers' costs, deter entry into the insurance market, and thus lead to higher prices for insurance or lower quality insurance. When an insurer with a large market share signs a contract including an MFN clause with a large hospital or physician group, that insurer has effectively increased its own costs and the costs of rival insurers and potential rivals in the insurance market. The MFN clause ensures that the hospital or physician group will not offer to provide services at lower fees to rival insurers or potential entrants. Thus, a large insurer getting most-favored-customer treatment may be able to charge prices above the competitive level or lower quality below the competitive level.

Alternative, noncollusive explanations for MFN contract clauses exist in the economics literature. MFN clauses may be a substitute for price discrimination or prices that decline over time (P'ng 1991). If heterogeneous insurers place different values on obtaining a contract with a particular hospital or physician group, then MFN clauses may allow the hospital or physician group to raise fees for "advance sales" to insurers who value the contract more highly and thus allow the providers to extract additional insurers' consumer surplus. Without MFN clauses, some high-valuation insurers might be willing to gamble on a price cut in future periods.

There are very important but very unsettled antitrust policy issues concerning MFN clauses in health care contracts. Court decisions have effectively established a rule of per se legality for MFN clauses (Bloch, Perlman, and Levasseur 1996), while the federal antitrust enforcement agencies have been challenging MFN clauses as anticompetitive and illegal.

Most courts considering the legality of MFN clauses between insurers and health care providers have upheld MFN clauses as not anticompetitive. In *Ocean State Physicians Health Plan v. Blue Cross/Blue*

Shield of Rhode Island,[23] the court found that the challenged MFN clause did not violate the antitrust laws and that the MFN clause had procompetitive effects, such as lowering the physician fees charged to Blue Cross/Blue Shield of Rhode Island. There was also, however, evidence presented in this case that suggested the MFN clause raised rival insurers' costs. The Blue Cross plan insisted on MFN clauses in its contracts with physicians who also contracted with Ocean State, a new HMO. Ocean State contracted with physicians on a 20 percent withhold basis, so physician payment rates depended on the profitability of the HMO. If Ocean State had a bad year, then Ocean State's physician payment rate was less than the Blue Cross payment rate. After Blue Cross insisted on MFN clauses, 350 of Ocean State's 1,200 physicians stopped providing services to Ocean State.

In *Blue Cross/Blue Shield v. Marshfield Clinic* it was alleged, among other things, that the Marshfield HMO had enforced its MFN clauses in contracts with physicians to facilitate collusion in the market for physician services and raise the prices of physician services. With respect to the argument that MFN clauses create a price floor for physician prices, Judge Posner said, "This is an ingenious but perverse argument. Most favored nation clauses are standard devices by which buyers try to bargain for low prices by getting the seller to agree to treat them as favorably as any of their other customers."[24]

More recently, however, the Federal Trade Commission and Department of Justice have successfully challenged MFN clauses used by dominant insurers as anticompetitive. In particular, the FTC and DOJ have argued that MFN clauses can lead to higher prices for health care services by facilitating horizontal coordination among health care providers. The agencies have argued that MFN clauses used by dominant insurers decrease health care providers' incentives to offer lower prices to other insurers and discourage selective discounting by providers. Second, the agencies have argued that MFN clauses may lead to higher prices for insurance by raising rival insurers' costs and deterring entry into the insurance market.

In February 1996, the DOJ filed an antitrust suit against Delta Dental of Rhode Island, the largest dental care insurer in Rhode Island,[25] for use of unlawful MFN clauses. The DOJ argued that use of MFN

23. 883 F.2d 1101 (1st Cir. 1989).

24. 65 F.3d at 1415.

25. About 90 percent of dentists in Rhode Island provide services to patients covered by Delta Dental of Rhode Island. Further, these dentists derive a significant portion of their revenue from treating these Delta patients (DOJ press release, 2/29/96).

clauses by Delta Dental of Rhode Island reduced price competition for dental services and made it more difficult for preferred provider organizations (PPOs) that could compete with Delta Dental to enter the insurance market, by making it harder for the PPOs to negotiate favorable fee schedules with dentists in Rhode Island. The court decided in favor of the DOJ. The DOJ challenged similar types of clauses against two other dental plans and one national vision care plan. These cases were settled out of court by the plans agreeing to discontinue the use of MFN contracts.

Conclusions

In this chapter we have considered the issues associated with the most common vertical restraints employed in health care markets. The use of these restraints is closely associated with managed care. As managed care has grown, so has the use of vertical restraints.

These restraints are a blessing in the sense that they have the potential to internalize externalities between doctors, hospitals, and insurers. They also represent a curse, in that they have the potential to be anticompetitive by foreclosing markets to rivals or facilitating collusion. Economic theory on the anticompetitive effects of vertical integration, exclusive dealing, and most-favored-nation clauses is far from conclusive. The most recent thinking on vertical restraints, the post–Chicago School, concludes that vertical restraints have the potential to be either efficiency enhancing or anticompetitive. Consequently, the merits of the employment of any vertical restraint must be judged individually, based on the assessed effects in that market.

We agree with this judgment. Unfortunately, that does not provide precise guidance about when vertical agreements are likely to be anticompetitive. It is our opinion that the two most important factors to assess are the possession of market power by firms involved in the vertical restraint and the difficulty of entry or expansion by rivals in the presence of the vertical restraint. This will require new thinking both on market definition under managed care and on the nature of barriers to entry under managed care.

References

Aghion, Phillippe, and Patrick Bolton. 1987. "Contracts as a Barrier to Entry." *American Economic Review* 77:388–401.

"Aligning Incentives: Contracting Strategies That Work for Providers and Plans." 1995. *Managed Care Week.* Special report.

American Medical News. 1996. 1:22–29.

Baker, Jonathan B. 1996. "Vertical Restraints with Horizontal Consequences: Competitive Effects of 'Most-Favored-Customer' Clauses." *Antitrust Law Journal* 64:517–34.

Bloch, Robert, Scott Perlman, and Luke Levasseur. 1996. "Most Favored Nation Clauses in Contracts between Health Care Networks and Providers: The Search for Practical Antitrust Guidance." *Antitrust Report* (September):3–10.

Bolton, Patrick, and Michael D. Whinston. 1993. "Incomplete Contracts, Vertical Integration, and Supply Assurance." *Review of Economic Studies* 60 (January):121–48.

Bork, Robert. 1978. *The Antitrust Paradox: A Policy at War with Itself.* New York: Basic Books.

Carlton, Dennis W., and Jeffrey M. Perloff. 1994. *Modern Industrial Organization,* 2d ed. New York: Harper Collins College Publishers.

Choi, Jay Pil, and San-Seung Yi. 1996. "Equilibrium Vertical Foreclosure with Investment." Unpublished manuscript, Columbia University.

Coase, R. 1937. "The Nature of the Firm." *Economica* 4:386–405.

Comanor, William S., and H. E. Frech III. 1985. "The Competitive Effects of Vertical Agreements." *American Economic Review* 75:539–46.

Cooper, Thomas. 1986. "Most-Favored-Customer Pricing and Tacit Collusion." *RAND Journal of Economics* 17(3):377–88.

Cooper, Thomas E., and Timothy L. Fries. 1991. "The Most-Favored-Nation Pricing Policy and Negotiated Prices." *International Journal of Industrial Organization* 9:209–23.

Corts, Kenneth S. 1996. "On the Competitive Effects of Price-Matching Policies." *International Journal of Industrial Organization* 15:283–99.

Department of Justice and Federal Trade Commission. 1996. Statements of Antitrust Enforcement Policy in Health Care, August.

Director, Aaron, and Edward H. Levi. 1956. "Law and the Future: Trade Regulation." *Northwestern University Law Review* 51:281–96.

Dranove, David D., and William D. White. 1996. "Specialization, Option Demand and the Pricing of Medical Services." *Journal of Economics and Management Strategy* 5:277–306.

———. 1997. "Emerging Issues in the Antitrust Definition of Healthcare Markets." *Electronic Health Economics Letters* 1 (5) (November):10–14.

Encinosa, William E. 1996. "Exclusive Contracting in Health Care Markets." Unpublished manuscript, University of Michigan.

Gal-Or, Esther. 1996. "Exclusionary Equilibria in Health Care Markets." *Journal of Economics and Management Strategy* 6 (Spring):5–43.

Gaynor, Martin. 1994. "Issues in the Industrial Organization of the Market for Physician Services." *Journal of Economics and Management Strategy* 3:211–55.

Gaynor, Martin, and Ching-to Albert Ma. 1996. "Insurance, Vertical Restraints, and Competition." Unpublished manuscript, Carnegie Mellon University.

Gillis, Kurt D., and David W. Emmons. 1993. "Physician Involvement with Alternative Delivery Systems." In Martin L. Gonzalez, ed., *Socioeconomic Characteristics of Medical Practice.* Chicago: American Medical Association.

Hart, Oliver, and Jean Tirole. 1990. "Vertical Integration and Market Foreclosure." *Brookings Papers on Economic Activity: Microeconomics*: 205–76.

Jensen, Gail A., Michael A. Morrisey, Shannon Gaffney, and Derek K. Liston. 1997. "The New Dominance of Managed Care: Insurance Trends in the 1990s." *Health Affairs* 16 (January–February):125–36.

Johnson, Julie. 1996. "Merger Spurs New Battle of Vicksburg." *American Medical News* 39, September 12:1, 28.

Katz, Michael L. 1989. "Vertical Contractual Relations." In Richard Schmalensee and Robert Willig, eds., *Handbook of Industrial Organization.* Amsterdam: North-Holland.

Klass, Michael W., and Michael A. Salinger. 1995. "Do New Theories of Vertical Foreclosure Provide Sound Guidance for Consent Agreements in Vertical Merger Cases?" *Antitrust Bulletin* 40 (Fall):667–98.

Krattenmaker, Thomas G., and Steven C. Salop. 1986a. "Competition and Cooperation in the Market for Exclusionary Rights." *American Economic Review*, Papers and Proceedings 76:109–13.

———. 1986b. "Anticompetitive Exclusion: Raising Rivals' Costs to Achieve Power over Price." *Yale Law Journal* 96:209–93.

Levin, Irving, and Associates. 1997. "Health Care Merger and Acquisition Report." *Modern Healthcare*, March 10:3.

Mathewson, G. Franklin, and Ralph A. Winter. 1987. "The Competitive Effects of Vertical Agreements: Comment." *American Economic Review* 77:1057–68.

Modern Healthcare. 1996, October 21:2.

———. 1997, March 10:22.

Ordover, Janusz A., Garth Saloner, and Steven C. Salop. 1990. "Equilibrium Vertical Foreclosure." *American Economic Review* 80:127–42.

P'ng, I. P. L. 1991. "Most-Favored-Customer Protection versus Price Discrimination over Time." *Journal of Political Economy* 99:1010–28.

Posner, Richard A. 1976. *Antitrust Law: An Economic Perspective.* Chicago: University of Chicago Press.

———. 1995. Opinion on *Blue Cross and Blue Shield United of Wisconsin and Compcare Health Services Insurance Corporation v. Marshfield Clinic and Security Health Plan of Wisconsin, Inc.*, U.S. Court of Appeals, Seventh Circuit, nos. 95–1965, 95–2140.

Rasmusen, Eric, J. Wiley, and M. Ramseyer. 1991. "Naked Exclusion." *American Economic Review* 81:1137–45.

Reiffen, David. 1992. "Equilibrium Vertical Foreclosure: Comment." *American Economic Review* 82:694–97.

Riordan, Michael H. 1996. "Anticompetitive Vertical Integration by a Dominant Firm." Unpublished manuscript, Boston University.

Riordan, Michael H., and Steven C. Salop. 1995. "Evaluating Vertical Mergers: A Post-Chicago Approach." *Antitrust Law Journal* 63:513–68.

Sage, William. 1997. "'Judge Posner's RFP: Antitrust Law and the Need for Better Research on Managed Care Markets." *Health Affairs* 16 (November–December):44–61.

Salinger, Michael A. 1988. "Vertical Mergers and Market Foreclosure." *Quarterly Journal of Economics* 103:335–56.

Salop, Steven C. 1986. "Practices That (Credibly) Facilitate Oligopoly Coordination." In J. Stiglitz and G. F. Mathewson, eds., *New Developments in the Analysis of Market Structure*. Cambridge, Mass.: MIT Press.

Salop, Steven C., and David T. Scheffman. 1983. "Raising Rivals' Costs." *American Economic Review*, Papers and Proceedings 73:267–71.

———. 1987. "Cost-Raising Strategies." *Journal of Industrial Economics* 36:19–34.

Schwartz, Marius. 1987. "The Competitive Effects of Vertical Agreements: Comment." *American Economic Review* 77:1063–68.

Spengler, Joseph J. 1950. "Vertical Integration and Antitrust Policy." *Journal of Political Economy* 53:347–52.

Vernon, John M., and Daniel A. Graham. 1971. "Profitability of Monopolization by Vertical Integration." *Journal of Political Economy* (July–August).

Westfield, Fred M. 1981. "Vertical Integration: Does Product Price Rise or Fall?" *American Economic Review* (June).

Williamson, Oliver. 1975. *Markets and Hierarchies: Analysis and Antitrust Implications*. New York: Free Press.

———. 1989. "Transaction Cost Economics." In Richard Schmalensee and Robert Willig, eds., *Handbook of Industrial Organization*. Amsterdam: North-Holland.

8

The Effects of Horizontal Hospital Mergers on Nonmerging Hospitals

Robert A. Connor and Roger D. Feldman

Merger activity in the health care sector has increased dramatically during the past decade, but there is strong disagreement over whether health care mergers benefit or harm consumers. Merger advocates believe that market consolidation is essential for eliminating duplicative services, reducing health care costs, and forming the integrated service networks that are required by today's health care consumers. They argue that price competition does not work in the health care sector as it does in other sectors. Competition advocates, in contrast, believe that market consolidation diminishes competition, increases prices, and reduces consumer welfare in the health care sector as well as in other sectors. They argue that hospital mergers are especially detrimental because of less mobile consumers and barriers to entry for providers (Blackstone and Fuhr 1989). Accordingly, the Federal Trade Commission and the Antitrust Division of the U.S. Department of Justice are increasingly scrutinizing hospital mergers, horizontal mergers in particular (Burda 1996).

In this chapter, we develop a framework to compare the effectiveness of different merger-related studies in measuring merger-related cost and price effects. We use this framework to summarize previous studies on horizontal hospital mergers. Then we present the results of an original large-scale empirical test of increased oligopoly power from horizontal hospital mergers that analyzes the effects of mergers on nonmerging hospitals in the same market area.

The authors appreciate support from AEI and the Agency for Health Care Policy and Research, as well as comments by an anonymous reviewer that prompted the merger and market-share interaction models. The views expressed and any errors are those of the authors.

164

TABLE 8–1
HYPOTHESIS TESTING COMPARING DIFFERENT SETS

Comparison	Can Test Hypotheses Concerning		Potential Bias in Testing $Cost_m$ and $Price_a$ from		
	$Cost_m$?	$Price_a$?	$Price_q$?	$Select_o$?	$Select_a$?
A vs. B	Yes	No	Yes	Yes	No
B vs. C	No	Yes	No	No	Yes
A vs. C	Yes	Yes	Yes	Yes	Yes
A vs. (B + C)	Yes	Mixed	Yes	Yes	Mixed
(A + B) vs. C	Mixed	Yes	Mixed	Mixed	Yes

SOURCE: Authors.

Methodological Framework

Our starting point is the trade-off in consumer welfare between merger-related cost savings from efficiencies and price increases from oligopoly power (Hay and Werden 1993; Stenbacka 1992). We generalize these concepts to include possible merger-related cost increases due to diseconomies of scale and merger implementation costs (Greene 1990; Kazemek 1991), merger-related price decreases if savings are passed on to consumers, and price changes due to merger-related quality changes and other product differentiation based on increased market share. A strong association between higher service volume and quality has been documented in the health care sector (Luft et al. 1986; Hughes et al. 1987). Broader geographic coverage from a merger may also be viewed as higher quality service. Price increases due to quality improvements need not decrease consumer welfare. Finally, we consider potential selection bias from unmeasured differences between merging versus nonmerging organizations and between areas with and without mergers. Below are listed the concepts that form the framework for comparing the studies of merger; table 8–1 illustrates methods:

- $Cost_m$: *Merger effects on merging organization's costs* may decrease costs through efficiencies or may increase costs through diseconomies of scale and merger implementation costs.
- $Price_a$: *Merger effects on prices of all organizations in the market area* may decrease prices if merger savings are passed on to consumers as lower prices, triggering nonmerging organizations in same market to reduce prices too, or may increase prices through oligopoly power.

165

- Price$_q$: *Merger effects on merging organization's prices because of quality or other product differentiation* may increase prices through improved quality (from increased service volume or broader geographic coverage) or other product differentiation following increased market share.
- Select$_o$: *Selection bias from unmeasured premerger characteristics of merging organizations,* which affect (changes in) merging organization cost or price.
- Select$_a$: *Selection bias from unmeasured premerger characteristics of market areas with mergers,* which affect (changes in) area cost or price.
- Organizational sets
  A: Merging organizations
  B: Nonmerging organizations ("rivals") in the same market area as merging organizations
  C: Nonmerging organizations in areas with no mergers

Table 8–1 specifies which comparisons test which merger effects as well as potential biases in these tests. Comparing merging organizations with nonmerging rivals (A versus B) can test for cost efficiencies but can be biased by unmeasured selection differences between merging and nonmerging organizations.

A comparison of nonmerging rivals versus organizations in areas without mergers (B versus C) can test for market price increases from oligopoly power. This comparison can be biased by unmeasured selection differences between areas with and without mergers, but is a cleaner test of oligopoly power than (A versus C), which includes quality effects on price and organizational selection bias in addition to area selection bias. Accordingly, (B versus C) comparisons are important for antitrust agencies and others concerned about possible merger-induced oligopoly power. This explains why we selected a B versus C design for this study.

Market Concentration

Most of what has been written on the effects of mergers of providers of health care has been derived from cross-sectional studies of the relationship between market concentration and hospital performance. The Herfindahl-Hirschman index (HHI), the sum of squared market share percentages for all firms in a market area, is often used as a measure of market concentration. Lower HHI values indicate greater market competition, higher values indicate greater market concentration, and an HHI of 10,000 is a monopoly.

The most common design for market concentration studies compares hospital performance in market areas with more hospitals (more competition, lower concentration, and lower HHI) to that of hospitals in areas with fewer hospitals (less competition, higher concentration, and higher HHI). Using the framework, these studies compare (A + B) versus C, with market concentration used as a proxy for merger to infer merger effects.

Studies of market concentration in health care that report higher costs (or prices) in areas with more hospitals are viewed as direct evidence that nonprice competition dominates health care markets and indirect evidence that hospital mergers produce cost savings from reduced service duplication. Nonprice competition in the health care sector has been called the "medical arms race," wherein competing hospitals acquire duplicative equipment and specialized services to attract physicians and patients. Nonprice competition can dominate a market when price-based competition is weak because of insurance-induced moral hazard, imperfect consumer information, or non-profit-maximizing organizations. In contrast, studies of market concentration in health care that report lower costs (or prices) in areas with more hospitals are generally viewed as direct evidence that price competition dominates health care markets and indirect evidence that hospital mergers increase prices (and costs) because of oligopoly power.

Using studies of market concentration to measure cost savings and price increases (from oligopoly power) can be biased by unmeasured selection differences between areas. Dranove, Shanley, and Simon (1992) noted that market areas with large populations tend to have more hospitals and also offer a wider range of expensive services. A study of market concentration that omits area population or an estimate of patient immigration may incorrectly attribute higher costs to greater competition. Measurement of oligopoly power through market concentration studies may also be biased by the effects of merger on quality that, in turn, affects price. Finally, measurement of both merger cost and price effects through such studies can be partly biased by unmeasured selection differences between merging and nonmerging hospitals.

The following studies of market concentration in health care provide evidence that health care markets were dominated by nonprice competition before the mid-1980s. Farley (1985), using counties as markets and data on 400 hospitals from 1970 to 1977, reported higher hospital costs per case in more competitive areas. Robinson and Luft (1985), using fifteen-mile radius circles as hospital markets and 1972 data, reported higher costs per day and per case in more competitive areas. Luft et al. (1986), using 1972 data for 3,584 community hospitals, found that hospitals with more neighboring hospitals offered more services. Robinson and Luft (1987), using twenty-four-kilometer circles

167

as hospital markets and 1982 data on 5,732 hospitals, reported a 26 percent higher cost per case in hospitals with more than 10 other hospitals within the circle than for those with no neighbors within the circle. Hughes and Luft (1991) reported that nonprice competition was more likely for specialized services than for primary care services.

Dranove, Shanley, and Simon (1992), however, reported minimal support for the medical arms race hypothesis in a study using 1983 hospital data. Noether (1988), using data for 1977–1978, also found evidence of both price and nonprice competition, but the net effect was insignificant. She noted that lack of an observed correlation between price and concentration could mean that the effects of price competition and quality competition cancel each other out. She concluded that, in spite of important distortions, price competition does operate in health care markets and would probably increase as these markets evolve.

Recent studies of concentration in health care markets have generally documented a shift away from dominance by nonprice competition to dominance by price-based competition. Longitudinal studies that analyze rates of cost and price inflation have provided the most support for this shift. Zwanziger and Melnick (1988) found higher hospital cost inflation in areas with more competing hospitals in California in the early 1980s, but this relationship disappeared in the mid-1980s. Melnick and Zwanziger (1988), using California hospital data from 1983 to 1985, reported 3.5 percent lower inflation rates for hospital cost per case in highly competitive markets.

Robinson and Luft (1988), using data from 1982–1986 for 5,490 hospitals, found lower cost inflation for hospitals in more competitive areas. Staten et al. (1988) found greater price discounts for a preferred provider organization (PPO) in areas with more competing hospitals. Melnick and Zwanziger (1989) measured discounts from charges, net patient revenue, gross charges, and costs in California hospitals from 1980 to 1987 and found lower inflation rates in more competitive areas. Zwanziger, Melnick, and Bamezai (1994) found larger reductions in hospital costs in more competitive areas of California from 1980 to 1990. Melnick et al. (1992), using 1987 data for 190 hospitals, reported that market competition led to lower PPO prices and that market concentration led to higher PPO prices. A decrease from three to two competitors was associated with a 9 percent price increase. They also noted that prices went up as the importance of a hospital to the PPO increased.

Dranove, Shanley, and White (1993), using 1983–1988 data for California hospitals, reported a shift to payer-driven competition, followed by falling margins and increasing conformity with the standard

168

industrial organization paradigm—increased competition leading to lower prices. According to their 1988 cross-sectional results, a three-to-two merger would increase an area's average price by 23 percent. Dranove et al. also noted that using list charges instead of actual prices biases results. Their observed relationships between higher competition and lower prices, for example, vanished when list charges were substituted for actual prices.

Recent studies of market concentration are not unanimous in their findings concerning market competition and costs. Manheim, Bazzoli, and Sohn (1994) reported that hospital markets with greater concentration had lower costs in 1988 as well as 1983. Lynk (1995a) also used the results of a cross-sectional analysis of 1989 hospital data to project that mergers of not-for-profit hospitals would reduce prices.

The results of studies of concentration in the health care market have been mixed, but most indicate a trend from dominance by non-price competition before the mid-1980s to dominance by price competition after the mid-1980s. This shift has been attributed to the Medicare Prospective Payment System (PPS), selective contracting by states, and greater market penetration by HMOs and other price-conscious payers (Dranove, Shanley, and White 1993).

Merger Performance

Longitudinal studies of merger performance compare organizational performance before with performance after a merger-related event. While studies of market concentration are used to infer merger effects from a cross-sectional association between market concentration and hospital performance, longitudinal performance studies measure merger effects directly from changes in merging organizations.

The most common design for these studies is comparison of pre- and postmerger organizational performance with that of a control group of nonmerging organizations during the same time period. These studies do not generally distinguish within the control group between nonmerging rival hospitals and hospitals in areas without mergers. Thus, using the framework, these studies generally compare A with (B + C). This comparison allows testing of merger-related cost savings from efficiencies and partial testing of price increases from oligopoly power. Tests using A versus (B + C) comparisons, however, can be biased by the effects of quality changes on price, unmeasured differences between merging and nonmerging organizations, and unmeasured differences between areas with and without mergers.

There have been a few large-scale longitudinal studies of merger performance of the health care sector. Mullner and Anderson (1987) analyzed the postmerger performance of sixty-two hospitals in thirty-two mergers identified by the American Hospital Association (AHA) during 1980–1985. Their premerger observation was one year before merger and their postmerger observation was one year after merger, except for financial ratios, which were measured up to four years after the merger. Comparison data for the industry were calculated for the midpoint of the study period and used as a control group. Mullner and Anderson reported higher occupancy rates for merged hospitals but no significant financial gains or losses.

Greene (1990) reported the results of a study of thirty-six hospitals in eighteen mergers from 1985 to 1987 that showed postmerger annual cost savings of 1–2 percent, as well as increased profits. Economies of scale were cited as the reason for savings. Average inflation for the industry was used as a control. Greene (1992) also reported postmerger cost savings in a study by Health Care Investment Analysts (HCIA) of fourteen hospitals from 1985 to 1990.

The U.S. Department of Health and Human Services (USDHHS 1992) studied eleven hospital mergers identified by the AHA for 1987 and compared their financial performance with eleven control hospitals that were geographically similar. This study also found modest merger-related cost savings. The AHA's Hospital Research and Educational Trust (HRET 1993) conducted a study of seventy-four hospital mergers from 1983 to 1988. They reported reduced acute-care services, decreased costs, and increased profits following the mergers.

Bogue et al. (1995) reported the results of a 1991 survey of sixty hospital mergers identified by the AHA from 1983 to 1988. They found that mergers were often followed by conversion of acute inpatient facilities to other functions. Lynk (1995b) documented case studies of postmerger cost savings from pooling staff and facilities for services with variable demand. Reduced standby capacity resulted in significant cost savings. Lynk noted that savings from reduced variability in demand through pooled services may be greater than savings from traditional economies of scale.

Alexander, Halpern, and Lee (1996) used data from the annual AHA surveys from 1980 to 1990 to compare the performance of ninety-two AHA identified mergers from 1982 to 1989 with the performance of a randomly selected control group. They measured the effects of mergers on scale (beds and adjusted admissions), efficiency (cost per adjusted admission and occupancy rate), and staffing (number of personnel). They reported that merged hospitals had a lower dollar amount increase in cost per adjusted admission and less decline in occupancy rate than hospitals in the control group. They also found that hospitals that merged after the implementation of the Medicare

PPS had greater efficiency gains than those hospitals that merged before PPS. Finally, they reported that mergers of similar sized hospitals had greater merger effects.

Connor, Feldman, and Dowd (1997) studied cost and price inflation for over 3,600 U.S. short-term general hospitals from 1986 to 1994, including over 244 hospitals in 122 mergers identified by the AHA. The study found postmerger reductions in cost and price per admission of approximately 5 percent relative to nonmerging hospitals. Merger-related cost savings and price reductions were much less, however, for mergers in highly concentrated markets.

To summarize, recent studies of merger performance of health care providers have generally reported modest cost savings for the merging organizations, although some evidence suggests that these cost savings vanish in more concentrated markets. Many of these studies either do not measure the effects of mergers on prices or report ambiguous price results. Among those studies that clearly report price effects, there is little evidence of large postmerger price increases and some evidence of postmerger price reductions.

Effects on Merger Rivals

The U.S. government's merger guidelines emphasize the importance of objective evidence concerning postmerger responses by competitors (Rill 1992; Baker 1988). A merger can lead to price increases if organizations either collude explicitly after merger or compete less strenuously because they realize that price reductions cause their rivals to reduce prices as well (Vistnes 1995). Accordingly, if mergers increase market prices through increased oligopoly power, then one would expect postmerger increases in the prices of rival organizations.

Most studies to date on the effects of mergers on rival organizations have not measured merger effects on rivals' prices or costs directly but rather attributed changes in rivals' stock prices to investor-anticipated changes in prices alone. These studies implicitly assume that merger-related savings from operating efficiencies affect only the costs of the merging organization, not those of its rivals. If premerger announcements (such as announcement of a planned merger) increase rivals' stock prices and antimerger announcements (such as FTC challenges) lower rivals' stock prices, then this is seen as evidence of merger-induced oligopoly power (Eckbo 1983; Perry and Porter 1985).

We know of only one study of the effects of health care mergers on rival organizations. Woolley (1989) measured the effects of twenty-nine merger-related events from 1969 to 1985 on the stock prices of rival hospital chains. He found that premerger announcements were followed by increases in rivals' stock prices and antimerger announcements were followed by decreases. Furthermore, the greater the impact of the merger on a local market, the greater the increase in a competitor's stock. Woolley concluded that mergers in the health care sector operate in a manner consistent with traditional oligopoly behavior. Higher concentration reduces rivalry, allowing both merging and nonmerging organizations to earn oligopoly profits.

Vita and Schumann (1991), however, criticized Woolley's study as including events that were too small to produce market power plausibly and as improperly identifying hospital chains as rivals when their hospitals did not overlap in local markets. Like Eckbo (1983, 1989), they suggested that the observed effects on rivals may be caused by the signal that rivals' assets are undervalued, not by oligopoly power.

There are also mixed views on the usefulness of studies of stock price in general for detecting merger effects on rivals. Woolley (1989) said that stock prices can measure merger effects better than profit margins, which are influenced by accounting methods. Werden and Williams (1989), however, wrote that evaluating merger effects through changes in stock prices is flawed because stock prices are noisy and crude signals. They note that aggregating data across many mergers may reduce noise but that it may also confound accurate measurement by lumping together the effects of collusive and efficient mergers.

Data

This study includes approximately 3,500 U.S. short-term general hospitals for which good longitudinal financial and statistical data are available for 1986 and 1994. To test the effects of merging hospitals on their nonmerging rivals, we identified nonmerging rivals and compared their performance with that of hospitals in areas without mergers. To ensure a clean (B versus C) comparison for measuring possible oligopoly power, we excluded the actual merging hospitals identified by the American Hospital Association from the analysis. The AHA defines a merger as two or more similar corporations coming together into a single surviving entity. Although any mergers not reported by the AHA remain in the control group and could have weakened measured effects, the control group is large, and AHA identification has been the standard method of identifying mergers in previous studies. Hospitals that were market area monopolies in 1986 were also excluded because they could not have become a rival of a merged hospital during this period. The resulting data set includes approximately two-thirds of the U.S. short-term general hospitals in operation during this entire period.

Of these, approximately one-third were nonmerging rivals in market areas with merging hospitals.

For defining hospital market areas, this study used the approximately 800 nonoverlapping, relatively self-contained Health Service Areas (HSAs) formed by Makuc et al. (1991) for the entire conterminous United States. Makuc et al. measured the flow of Medicare hospital stays between counties, used cluster analysis to identify counties linked by high border crossing, and combined linked counties to form HSAs. The median number of counties per HSA is three, and the median number of hospitals per HSA is five. Makuc et al. also studied the degree to which patients traveled outside the market area for care and estimated the percentage of outmigration for each area. Makuc's HSAs were used exclusively because they are empirically based on patient travel patterns, they include measures of fringe supply (HSA border crossing), counties are generally thought to be too small for rural hospital market areas, and we are not aware of alternative non-overlapping hospital market areas for the entire nation. County demographic, economic, and other data came from the Bureau of Health Profession's 1994 Area Resource File and were combined into HSAs to serve as market area variables (USDHHS/ARF 1994).

Financial and statistical data came from the Health Care Financing Administration PPS data sets after editing to ensure data quality (HCFA 1986–1994). Editing strategies included reversing erroneous negative allowances and rejecting hospitals with no allowances, cross-sectional comparison of related information from different sections of the Medicare cost report to check internal consistency, cross-sectional comparison with related information in corresponding records in the AHA data sets, and longitudinal review of financial and statistical data to identify abrupt and possibly erroneous changes. Data on hospital characteristics and merger identification came from the AHA Annual Hospital Surveys (AHA 1986–1994). Data on HMO penetration rates came from the work of Douglas Wholey at Carnegie Mellon University. Area wage indexes and case mix indexes came from HCFA (HCFA 1994).

Methods

Our basic study design is B versus C—comparing the performance of nonmerging rivals of merging hospitals with that of hospitals in areas without mergers, during the 1986–1994 time period in which the mergers occurred. It differs from Woolley's study in several respects. First, actual changes in costs and prices were measured over several years instead of inferring future prices from short-term changes in stock

173

price. Second, hospitals classified as rivals were all located in the same empirically defined market areas as the merging hospitals. Third, more than a thousand observations of the effects of actual mergers on rivals were measured, in comparison with twenty-nine observations of the effects of merger-related announcements on rivals. Finally, the data set covers mergers during the most recent decade.

Operating expenses and revenues were used instead of total expenses and total revenues to focus on hospitals' core business of patient care, rather than on endowment size or nonoperating subsidies. Net patient revenue was used instead of gross charges because prices actually paid have more economic meaning than "list" prices (Dranove, Shanley, and White 1993). Bivariate comparisons of the differences in area and organizational characteristics between merger rivals and hospitals in areas without mergers were drawn in addition to the full multivariate analyses.

Before developing the longitudinal multivariate models, we had to specify the underlying cross-sectional models. We developed cross-sectional models for average hospital operating expense per admission, average patient revenue (charges minus allowances) per admission, and operating profit ratio (patient revenues divided by operating expenses) for the 1986 premerger period. As done by Robinson and Luft (1988), admissions were used as the primary measure of hospital output in the average cost models, reflecting the emphasis on payment per admission such as in Medicare's Prospective Payment System. Hospital days and the percentage of outpatient to total charges were included on the right-hand side of the models to adjust for intensity of service per admission and recognize non-inpatient hospital outputs. The White (1980) covariance estimator was used to correct heteroskedasticity in least-squares estimation and obtain more accurate significance levels for variable coefficients in all models.

Following Robinson and Phibbs (1989) and Breyer (1987), we began with a modified constant elasticity function for total hospital cost as shown in equation 8–1. Only one direct price input, an area wage index, was used because much of hospital expenses are wages and markets for equipment and supplies are less local than those for labor. The following indirect factors, which are thought to influence average cost or revenue, were also included: percentages of Medicare days, Medicaid days, and disproportionate share payments; index of case mix; percentage of special care and subacute care days; occupancy rate; and percentage of capital costs.

In addition to price and output factors, hospital and market area factors from the literature that are thought to refine output measurement, influence hospital production functions, and affect hospital revenues were also included as regressors. Binary cost or price-shifting factors included for-profit ownership and Council of Teaching Hospitals (COTH) membership. Market factors included as continuous variables were area HHI, physicians per capita, area IPA and group HMO penetration, total population, per capita income, unemployment rate, percentage of elderly, percentage of young women, percentage of white-collar workers, percentage of manufacturing workers, unemployment rate, market area size, percentage of patient area outmigration, census division dummy variables, and market area urban-rural (0–9) designation. Inclusion of a variable for patient outmigration is unusual, but measurement of border crossing for care and "fringe demand" is important in analysis of health care markets (Dranove et al. 1992).

$$C_{it} = e^{\alpha t} e^{\Sigma f \beta 1 f X itf} (\pi_f P_{itf}{}^{\beta 2f}) Q_{it}{}^{\beta 3} (\pi_f V_{itf}{}^{\beta 4f}) (\pi_f A_{itf}{}^{\beta 5f}) e^{uit} \qquad (8\text{–}1)$$

where, C_{it} = total cost for hospital (i); $\beta._f$ = estimated model coefficients; Σ_f = sum of (f) factors; π_f = product of (f) factors; α_t = general period factor affecting all hospitals; X_{itf} = binary factors: $f = 1, \ldots, 2$: for-profit hospital and COTH teaching hospital membership; P_{itf} = input prices and other cost and price influencing factors: $f = 1, \ldots,$ 9: area wage index; percentage of Medicare, percentage of Medicaid, percentage of disproportionate share payments, case mix index, percentage of subacute days, hospital occupancy, and percentage of capital cost; Q_{it} = admissions; V_{itf} = outputs other than admissions: $f = 1, \ldots, 2$: days, outpatient services; A_{itf} = market area factors: area HHI, physicians per capita, IPA and group HMO penetration, total population, per capita income, unemployment rate, percentage of elderly, percentage of young women, percentage of white-collar workers, percentage of manufacturing workers, area size, percentage of patient outmigration, census divisions, and urban-rural code.

As suggested by Kmenta (1986), higher-order output and price terms and interactions were also estimated, but the F-test associated with the higher-order terms was insignificant, so we retained the form in equation 8–1 for the virtue of simplicity. To reduce heteroskedasticity, we divided both sides of equation 8–1 by admissions (Q_{it}) to get the average cost per admission model given in equation 8–2:

$$AC_{it} = C_{it}/Q_{it} = e^{\alpha t} e^{\Sigma f \beta 1 f X itf} (\pi_f P_{itf}{}^{\beta 2f}) Q_{it}{}^{\beta 3 - 1} (\pi_f V_{itf}{}^{\beta 4f}) (\pi_f A_{itf}{}^{\beta 5f}) e^{uit}. (8\text{–}2)$$

To reduce multicollinearity, Robinson and Phibbs (1989) and Breyer (1987) have recommended dividing each $V_{itf}{}^{\beta 4f}$ term by $Q_{it}{}^{\beta 4f}$. The equation remains balanced by multiplying the admissions term (Q_{it}) by $Q_{it}{}^{\Sigma f \beta 4f}$. The result is equation 8–3:

175

$$AC_{it} = C_{it}/Q_{it}$$

$$= e^{\alpha t}e^{\Sigma f\beta 1fXitf}(\pi_f P_{itf}{}^{\beta 2f})Q_{it}{}^{\beta 3-1+\Sigma f\beta 4f}(\pi_f(V_{itf}/Q_{it})^{\beta 4f})(\pi_f A_{itf}{}^{\beta 5f})e^{uit}. \quad (8\text{--}3)$$

So that this model can be estimated as a linear function, we took the natural log of both sides, yielding equation 8–4:

$$lnAC_{it} = \alpha_t + \Sigma_f\beta_{1f}X_{itf} + \Sigma_f\beta_{2f}lnP_{itf} + (\beta_3 - 1 + \Sigma_f\beta_{4f})lnQ_{it}$$

$$+ \Sigma_f\beta_{4f}ln(V_{itf}/Q_{it}) + \Sigma_f\beta_{5f}lnA_{itf} + u_{it}. \quad (8\text{--}4)$$

Our next step was to use the cross-sectional model in equation 8–4 to develop a longitudinal model with which to estimate the effects of hospital mergers on changes in rival hospitals' average costs, average revenues, and profit ratios from 1986 to 1991. To have each hospital serve as its own control, we used a first-difference model for the change in average cost per admission from period t to $t + 1$ as shown in equation 8–5 wherein: $\triangle\ lnAC_i = lnAC_{it+1} - lnAC_{it}$ and other $\triangle$ variables are similarly defined first differences.

Binary variables were subtracted in the change model. This assumes, for example, that a change from for-profit to not-for-profit status has an impact that is equal and opposite to a change in the other direction and that remaining for-profit has the same impact as remaining not-for-profit. With the exception of area population, market factors for which both pre- and postperiod data were available were included in the longitudinal model as change values, and the rest were included as constant values. Area population was included as both a baseline constant and a change variable because Dranove, Shanley, and Simon (1992) noted that it is probably correlated with unmeasured market variables (for example, travel time, market structure, or buyer coalitions).

For the longitudinal models measuring the effects of mergers on rival hospitals, two independent variables were tested in separate models. The first is a binary variable with a value of 1 for hospitals in areas with a merger and 0 for hospitals in areas without a merger. Since Schumann (1993) stressed the importance of the size of the merging organization in the local market to the effects on rival organizations, the second variable measures the relative importance of the merger to the nonmerging rival. The relative importance of the merger was measured by the percentage of 1986 adjusted admissions in the market area that were involved in the merger. These measures were made to interact with organizational and market variables such as HHI, baseline occupancy, and rural versus urban area in separate models.

Terms representing having one's neighbor merge between time t and $t + 1$ were added to the first difference model because they represent a change in hospital characteristics that occurred during this period. In the binary longitudinal model shown in equation 8–5, a binary rival variable (Mi) is added.

$$\triangle\, lnAC_i = \triangle\alpha + \Sigma_f\beta_{1f}\triangle X_{if} + \Sigma_f\beta_{2f}\triangle lnP_{if}$$

$$+ (\beta_3 - 1 + \Sigma_f\beta_{4f})\triangle\, lnQ_i + \Sigma_f\beta_{4f}\triangle ln(V_{if}/Q_{it})$$

$$+ \Sigma_f\beta_{5f}\triangle\, lnA_{lif} + \Sigma_f\beta_{6f}lnA_{2if} + \beta_7 lnM_i + \triangle\, u_i. \qquad (8\text{–}5)$$

As noted by Robinson and Phibbs (1989), however, equation 8–5 is biased if cost levels in the base year are affected by disturbances correlated with being in an area in which a merger occurs. If hospitals in areas that spawn mergers tended to have initially lower costs, then equation 8–5 will underestimate merger effects. If hospitals in areas that spawn mergers tend to have initially higher costs, then equation 8–5 will overestimate merger effects. This may be viewed as a selection bias problem with respect to unmeasured cost-increase-influencing characteristics that differ between areas with and areas without mergers. As discussed by Robinson and Phibbs, the simplest way to model the impact of these disturbances on cost increases is to assume that the error term in equation 8–5 is generated by a first-order autoregressive process:

$$u_{it+1} = pu_{it} + \epsilon_{it+1}, 0<p<1. \qquad (8\text{–}6)$$

Accordingly, one can control for area selection bias by including the estimated residuals from the base period cross-sectional model ($\hat{u}_{it}$) in the change model. Specifically, one substitutes $(p\text{-}1)\hat{u}_{it} + \epsilon_{it+1}$ for $\triangle u_i$ in equation 8–5, yielding equation 8–7.

$$\triangle\, lnAC_i = \triangle\, \alpha + \Sigma_f\beta_{1f}\triangle X_{if} + \Sigma_f\beta_{2f}\triangle lnP_{if}$$

$$+ (\beta_3 - 1 + \Sigma_f\beta_{4f})\triangle lnQ_i + \Sigma_f\beta_{4f}\triangle ln(V_{if}/Q_{it})$$

$$+ \Sigma_f\beta_{5f}\triangle\, lnA_{lif} + \Sigma_f\beta_{6f}lnA_{2if} + \beta_7 M_i + (p-1)\hat{u}_{it} + \epsilon_{it+1}. \qquad (8\text{–}7)$$

In our previous study of the effects of mergers on the merging hospitals themselves, we used a reduced-form longitudinal model without changes in occupancy or HHI to measure merger effects because changes in occupancy are a major avenue for merger efficiencies to occur and changes in HHI are a major avenue for oligopoly power to occur. Conceptually, including these variables would have overcontrolled when measuring merger effects, so we omitted them in the main merger models. We did empirically test the models with these variables included anyway and the results were not significantly changed. To maintain the same basic model for this study, we also excluded these two change variables in the longitudinal models measuring merger effects on rivals.

Results

Preliminary, bivariate comparisons of area and hospital characteristics for merger rival hospitals as opposed to hospitals within areas without mergers are given in table 8–2. Approximately one-third of the hospitals were in areas with AHA-identified mergers. Market areas of merger rivals generally had greater competition (lower HHI), higher HMO penetration, more physicians per capita, larger populations, higher per capita incomes and wage indexes, and more urbanization than those of hospitals in areas without mergers. Table 8–2 also shows differences in hospital characteristics between merger rival hospitals and hospitals in areas without mergers. The percentages of for-profit and COTH hospitals were higher among merger rivals. Merger rivals also tended to have more beds and higher admissions and occupancy rates than hospitals in areas without mergers. Because of the increasing importance of outpatient services, we made an adjustment to reflect outpatient services for use in these simple bivariate comparisons. Net patient revenue and operating expenses were multiplied times the percentage of (inpatient)/(total charges) before division by admissions to get revenues and expenses per outpatient-adjusted admission. Merger rivals had higher average net revenue per outpatient-adjusted admission in both 1986 ($3,532 versus $2,871) and 1994 ($5,618 versus $4,846) compared with hospitals in areas without mergers, but this gap narrowed from 1986 to 1994. In 1986, merger rival prices were 23 percent higher those of hospitals in areas without mergers, but by 1994 they were only 16 percent higher. Thus, simple bivariate comparison does not suggest price increases for merger rivals.

The results of the 1994 cross-sectional models for average cost, average price, and operating margin for all hospitals in the data set (which excludes those that merged and market area monopolies) are shown in table 8–3. The F-tests for these models are extremely significant and the R-squared values show that these models explain over 60 percent of the interhospital variation in cost and price per admission. The coefficients on area HHI for the cost and price models are positive but marginally insignificant. Since the HHI coefficients were negative and significant in the 1986 cross-sectional model (not shown), however, this sign reversal is additional evidence of a shift away from nonprice competition during this decade. This confirmatory evidence is particularly useful because it is obtained by using the same cross-sectional model on the same data set for two observations that are a decade

TABLE 8–2
AREA AND HOSPITAL CHARACTERISTICS OF MERGER RIVAL
HOSPITALS AND NONRIVALS

Characteristic	Merger Rivals (A)	Nonrivals (B)	(A–B)/B (%)
Number of observations	1,203	2,423	
Mean area characteristics			
Herfindahl index (HHI) 1986	987	2,229	−56■
HMO penetration 1987, %	13.9	7.9	76■
Group HMO pen. 1987, %	8.8	4.6	91■
MDs per 10,000 people 1986	20.5	15.4	33■
Population (thous.) 1986	2,490	1,051	137■
Per capita income 1986, $	15,542	13,475	15■
Wage index 1986	10,940	9,828	11■
Urban-rural code (0–9) 1991	1.6	3.5	−55■
Mean hospital characteristics			
For-profit ownership 1986, %	14.4	11.1	29■
COTH teaching hospital 1986, %	13.1	6.3	109■
Beds 1986	262	194	35■
Admissions 1986	8,616	6,199	39■
Length of stay 1986	7.5	7.8	−4
% occupancy 1986	57.2	51.8	10■
% special care days 1986	7.0	5.7	23■
% subacute days 1986	15.5	18.2	−15■
% Medicare hospital days 1986	45.2	46.6	−3■
% Medicaid hospital days 1986	8.8	9.0	−1
% outpatient/total charges 1986	20.3	21.2	−4■
% disproportionate share 1986	0.6	.40	56■
% capital/total expenses 1986	10.1	9.9	2
Case mix index 1986	1.1754	1.1263	4■
Net pt. revenue (000$) 1986	42,233	26,385	60■
Net pt. revenue (000$) 1994	80,041	51,722	55■
REV per admission 1986, $	4,406	3,633	21■
REV per admission 1994, $	8,499	7,755	10■
REV per output-adjusted adm. 1986, $	3,532	2,871	23■
REV per output-adjusted adm. 1994, $	5,618	4,846	16■
Operating exps. (000$) 1986	42,613	26,424	61■

(Table continues)

TABLE 8-2 (continued)

Characteristic	Merger Rivals (A)	Nonrivals (B)	(A–B)/B (%)
Operating exps. (000$) 1994	81,263	51,701	57■
EXP per admission 1986, $	4,474	3,717	20■
EXP per admission 1994, $	8,650	7,878	10■
EXP per output-adjusted adm. 1986, $	3,579	2,930	22■
EXP per output-adjusted adm. 1994, $	5,699	4,902	16■
REV/EXP ratio 1986	0.991	0.981	1**
REV/EXP ratio 1994	0.993	0.993	−0

NOTE: Single t-test significance: * = $p<.01$ ** = $p<.001$ ■ = $p<.0001$.
SOURCE: Authors.

apart. As we will see, it is also confirmed by the results of the longitudinal model.

The coefficients on for-profit ownership and COTH teaching hospital status indicate that, other things being equal, costs for for-profit hospitals were 8 percent lower and costs for COTH hospitals were 25 percent higher. The .46 coefficient on the area wage index appears reasonable in light of the theoretical expectation that it should approximate the percentage of hospital operating expenses for personnel. The 1.02 coefficient for the index of case mix is quite close to 1.00, indicating that it is an excellent measure of the impact of case mix on costs. A 10 percent increase in the index of case mix, for example, would be associated with almost exactly a 10 percent increase in cost. This is evidence that the case mix weights are not compressed.

As one would expect, table 8–3 shows that increased special care days increase costs (and prices) and that increased subacute days decrease costs (and prices). Higher occupancy reduces average cost because of more efficient use of fixed assets. The significant positive coefficient on admissions (measuring the effect of squared admissions in this average cost model) provides evidence of economies of scale. Hospitals in areas with greater penetration by IPA-type and group-type HMOs have lower costs and prices, but, consistent with the literature on HMO price shopping, the reductions caused by group-type HMOs are stronger than those by IPA-type HMOs (Kralewski et al. 1992).

Table 8–4 shows the results of the multivariate model for average

TABLE 8–3
MODELS FOR LOGS OF EXPENSE PER ADMISSION, REVENUE PER
ADMISSION, AND REVENUE TO EXPENSE, 1994

Variable and Coefficient	Log of Expense/ Admission	Log of Revenue/ Admission	Log of Revenue/ Expense
Constant	−.0763	.5953	.6717≈
Log area Herfindahl index 1994	.0195~	.0176~	−.0020
For-profit status 1994 (1 = yes)	−.0827■	.0057	.0884■
COTH teaching hosp. 1994 (1 = yes)	.2490■	.1965■	−.0526■
Log area wage index 1994	.4647■	.4954■	.0307~
Log % Medicare 1994	−.0211	.0253	.0464■
Log % Medicaid 1994	−.0192*	−.0146≈	.0047
Log % disproportionate share 1994	.0112≈	.0047	−.0065*
Log case mix index 9/94	1.02■	1.04■	.0159
Log % special care days 1994	.0375■	.0413■	.0038
Log % subacute days 1994	−.0233■	−.0184■	.0048*
Log % occupancy 1994	−.1875■	−.1263■	.0612■
Log admissions 1994	−.0625■	−.0412■	.0213■
Log length of stay 1994	.3554■	.3247■	−.0307■
Log % outpatient/total charges	.2852■	.2976■	.0124≈
Log % capital cost 1994	.0782■	.0834■	.0052
Log area MDs/10,000 1994	−.0162	−.0032	.0130~
Log area % IPA HMO members 1994	−.0055	−.0093≈	−.0038≈
Log area % group HMO members 1994	−.0174■	−.0165■	.0009
Log area population 1994	.0076	.0028	−.0048
Log area per capita income 1994	.2486■	.1448■	−.1038■
Log area unemployment rate 1992	.0894■	.0420*	−.0474■

(Table continues)

181

TABLE 8-3 (continued)

Variable and Coefficient	Log of Expense/ Admission	Log of Revenue/ Admission	Log of Revenue/ Expense
Log area % people over 65 in 1990	−.0021	−.0470	−.0449*
Log area % women 15–44 in 1990	.2653≈	.1859~	−.0794~
Log area % white collar 1990	.0899	.0657	−.0242
Log area % manuf. workers 1990	−.0218~	−.0128	.0090~
Log area size (sq. mi.)	.0138≈	.0135≈	−.0003
Log area % outmigration	−.0082	−.0050	.0033
New England[a]	.0607■	.0669■	.0062
East north central[b]	.0830■	.1107■	.0277■
East south central[c]	.0087	.0369■	.0282■
West south central[d]	−.0016	−.0014	.0002
West mountain[e]	.0408≈	.0684■	.0275*
West Pacific[f]	.0265	.0494*	.0229*
Log area urban-rural (0–9) code	.0100	.0026	−.0073
Sample characteristics Number of			
observations	3617	3617	3617
Dependent var. mean	8.92	8.91	−.0101
R-squared	.6079	.6101	.2854
F-test (34, 3582)	163.37	164.88	42.07
F-test significance	.0000	.0000	.0000

NOTE: Coefficient significance: ~ p<.1 ≈ p<.05 * p<.01 ■ p<.001.
a. Maine, Vermont, New Hampshire, Connecticut, Rhode Island.
b. Ohio, Missouri, Indiana, Illinois, Wisconsin.
c. Kentucky, Tennessee, Mississippi, Alabama.
d. Arkansas, Louisiana, Texas, Oklahoma.
e. Montana, Wyoming, Colorado, New Mexico, Arizona, Utah.
f. Washington, Oregon, California, Alaska, Hawaii.
SOURCE: Authors.

cost and price inflation from 1986 to 1994, including a binary variable with a value of 1.0 for merger rivals. Overall, these models are very significant, explaining approximately 60 percent of interhospital differences in cost and price inflation from 1986 to 1994. The coefficient for the binary merger rival variable in the price inflation model (.000678)

TABLE 8–4

EFFECTS OF HOSPITAL MERGER ON THE CHANGE IN LOGS OF EXPENSE PER
ADMISSION, REVENUE PER ADMISSION, AND REVENUE TO EXPENSE OF
NONMERGING RIVALS, 1986–1994

Variable and Coefficient	△ Log of Expense/ Admission	△ Log of Revenue/ Admission	△ Log of Revenue/ Expense
Constant	.3791	.2681	− .0273
Merger in hospital's market	.0012	.0007	− .0032
Log area Herfindahl index 1986	.0350■	.0389■	.0014
△ For-profit status	− .0321	.0340	.0773■
△ COTH teaching hospital	.0768■	.0634■	− .0217≈
△ Log area wage index	.2432■	.3581■	.1112■
△ Log % Medicare	.0625■	.0699■	.0183≈
△ Log % Medicaid	.0121≈	.0114≈	− .0005
△ Log % dispropor- tionate share	− .0103*	− .0125■	− .0037~
△ Log case mix index	.2843■	.3266■	.0274
△ Log % special care days	.0347■	.0271■	− .0060~
△ Log % subacute days	− .0153■	− .0151■	.0003
△ Log admissions	− .4204■	− .3289■	.0880■
△ Log length of stay	.2009■	.2215■	.0195■
△ Log % outpatient charges	.1101■	.0971■	− .0107~
△ Log % capital cost	.0851■	.0657■	− .0179■
△ Log area MDs/ 10,000	.1020*	.0787≈	− .0042
△ Log % open HMO members	.0145≈	.0183*	.0047
△ Log % IPA HMO members	.0002	− .0044	− .0047*
△ Log % group HMO members	− .0074~	− .0124*	− .0037~
△ Log area popula- tion	.2717■	.2435■	.0071
△ Log area per capita income	.1589≈	.1570≈	− .0367

(Table continues)

TABLE 8-4 (continued)

Variable and Coefficient	△ Log of Expense/ Admission	△ Log of Revenue/ Admission	△ Log of Revenue/ Expense
△ Log area unemployment rate	−.0065	−.0464≈	−.0580■
Log area population 1986	−.0140	−.0126	.0026
Log area % people over 65 1990	−.0498~	−.0555~	−.0058
Log area % women 15–44 1990	.0337	.0791	.0404
Log area % white collar 1990	−.0007	−.0217	−.0297
Log area % manuf. workers 1990	.0136	.0035	−.0121≈
Log area size (sq. mi.)	.0085	.0133≈	.0023
Log area % outmigration	.0031	.0188~	.0168■
New England[a]	.0026	.0178	.0241*
East north central[b]	−.0078	.0071	.0098≈
East south central[c]	−.0396■	−.0248≈	.0166*
West south central[d]	−.0472■	−.0497*	−.0019
West mountain[e]	−.0333~	−.0277	.0067
West Pacific[f]	−.0841■	−.0775■	.0072
Log area urban-rural (0–9) code	.0446*	.0483*	.0029
Residual from 1986 model	−.4022■	−.4527■	−.7132■
Number of observations	3328	3328	3328
Dependent var. mean	.7670	.7804	.0134
R-squared	.6126	.5751	.4330
F-test (37, 3290)	140.59	120.37	67.91
F-test significance	.0000	.0000	.0000

NOTE: Coefficient significance: ~ p<.1   ≈ p<.05   * p<.01   ■ p<.001.
a. Maine, Vermont, New Hampshire, Connecticut, Rhode Island.
b. Ohio, Missouri, Indiana, Illinois, Wisconsin.
c. Kentucky, Tennessee, Mississippi, Alabama.
d. Arkansas, Louisiana, Texas, Oklahoma.
e. Montana, Wyoming, Colorado, New Mexico, Arizona, Utah.
f. Washington, Oregon, California, Alaska, Hawaii.
SOURCE: Authors.

is small and not statistically significant ($p = .94237$), providing no evidence of price increases for merger rivals. The coefficient for baseline 1986 HHI (.038924) in the price inflation model is positive and highly significant ($p = .00037$), providing additional evidence of a shift away from nonprice competition in health care markets since the mid-1980s. Areas with higher 1986 HHI had higher cost and price inflation from 1986 to 1994. This finding confirms the trends reported by Zwanziger and Melnick (1988), Robinson and Luft (1988), and Dranove, Shanley, and Simon (1993).

Table 8–5 shows three alternative longitudinal models of the effects of hospital mergers on nonmerging rivals in the same market area. The HHI interaction model measures whether the effect on merger rivals is different in areas with an HHI over 2,000, but neither the merger rival variable nor the HHI interaction variable is statistically significant.

The linear merger market share model measures whether the effect on merger rivals depends, in a linear manner, on the market power of the merging hospitals. The market power of the merging hospitals is measured by the percentage of a market area's total adjusted admissions involved in the merger. It is zero for hospitals in areas without mergers. Increased market power from large mergers could cause the merging organizations to "dominate" the market and suppress the prices of rival organizations, particularly if there are merger-related quality improvements or other forms of product differentiation (McGuckin, Warren-Boulton, and Waldstein 1992).

The results of the linear merger market share model in the price inflation model show a marginally significant ($p = .04730$) positive coefficient (.049619) for the binary merger rival variable and a marginally significant ($p = .03552$) negative coefficient ($-.015905$) for the percentage of area admissions involved in the merger. These results suggest that smaller mergers (under 20 percent of market area admissions) are associated with modest (1–3 percent) increases in rivals' prices and that larger mergers (over 20 percent of market areas admissions) are associated with modest (1–2 percent) decreases in rivals' prices. Closer investigation of the relationship between merger size and rivals' prices, however, suggested that the relationship is not a linear one, so a nonlinear model was estimated. In the nonlinear merger market share model, merger rivals were divided into three approximately equal groups: rivals of mergers involving 1–7 percent of market admissions, rivals of mergers involving 7+ percent to 19 percent of market admissions, and rivals of mergers involving 19+ percent of market admissions. The results of this model provide significant ($p = .01884$) evidence of modest (3 percent) increases in

TABLE 8–5

ALTERNATIVE MODELS FOR CHANGE IN LOGS OF EXPENSE PER
ADMISSION, REVENUE PER ADMISSION, AND REVENUE TO EXPENSE,
1986–1994

Dependent Variable	△ Log of Expense/ Admission	△ Log of Revenue/ Admission	△ Log of Revenue/ Expense
HHI interaction model			
Merger in hospital's market	− .0090	− .0084	− .0026
Market merger × HHI > 2000	.0179	.0139	− .0017
HHI 1986 > 2000 (1 = yes)	.0147	.0245 ≈	.0081 ~
:			
Linear merger market share model			
Merger in hospital's market	.0406 ~	.0496 ≈	.0094
Log % admissions merged in			
market	− .0128 ~	− .0159 ≈	− .0041
:			
Nonlinear merger market share model			
1% to 7% admissions merged in			
market	.0030	.0060	.0027
7 + % to 19% admissions merged			
in market	.0347*	.0331 ≈	− .0041
19 + % admissions merged in			
market	− .0151	− .0161	− .0045
:			

: = results for other variables were similar to those in longitudinal model in
table 8–4 and are not repeated here.
NOTE: Coefficient significance: ~ $p<.01$ ≈ $p<.05$ * $p<.01$ ▪ $p<.001$.
SOURCE: Authors.

prices for rivals of mergers involving 7 + percent to 19 percent of market area admissions but no statistically significant evidence of effects
for rivals of smaller or larger mergers.

Conclusion

The first main finding of this study is the general lack of large, statistically significant effects of hospital mergers on the prices of rivals in the
same market areas. The one exception is a 3 percent price increase for
rivals in areas with mergers involving 7 + to 19 percent of the area's

adjusted admissions. An explanation for this result is as follows. Small mergers (1–7 percent of area admissions) are not large enough to increase oligopoly power significantly in the market and do not have much influence on rivals' prices. Medium-sized mergers (7–19 percent) result in modest oligopoly power, which rivals use to increase their prices slightly. Larger mergers result in market domination by the merging organizations, which suppresses the prices of nonmerging rivals. For price differences based on market domination to work in the long run, they must be accompanied by quality improvements or other forms of product differentiation for the merging organizations. In light of these results, we would advise policy makers not to assume that horizontal health care mergers cause increased market area prices through oligopoly power unless such price increases are documented by future large-scale longitudinal studies.

The second main finding is confirmation of a shift away from non-price competition in health care markets since the mid-1980s. This finding is based on: reversal of the negative coefficient on area HHI from 1986 to 1994 in the cross-sectional cost and price models, and the significant positive coefficients for 1986 HHI in the longitudinal models of hospital cost and price inflation from 1986 to 1994. The medical arms race model appears to be less relevant to health care markets today than it was a decade ago.

The limitations to this study could be addressed in future research. First, although the study is large compared with previous studies and AHA identification has been the standard method of identifying mergers, it would be valuable to conduct larger-scale studies that include all hospital mergers, not just those identified by changing AHA ID numbers. Second, although we included the percentages of Medicare and Medicaid volume among the control variables and also found no significant interactions between those percentages and merger-to-rival effects, future studies should investigate more closely the relationships among market competition, market-driven versus publicly regulated prices, and cost shifting. Finally, we recommend additional research into the probably nonlinear relationships among HHI, the market share of merging organizations, and the effects of mergers on costs and prices. This recommendation applies to both merging organizations and their within-market rivals.

References

Alexander, Jeffrey A., Michael T. Halpern, and Shoou-Yih Lee. 1996. "The Short-Term Effect of Merger on Hospital Operations." *Health Services Research* 30(6):827–47.

American Hospital Association. 1986–1994. *Annual Survey of Hospitals* (data set). Chicago: AHA.

Baker, Jonathan B. 1988. "The Antitrust Analysis of Hospital Mergers and the Transformation of the Hospital Industry." *Law and Contemporary Problems* 51(2):93–164.

Blackstone, Erwin A., and Joseph P. Fuhr Jr. 1989. "Hospital Mergers and Antitrust: An Economic Analysis." *Journal of Health Politics, Policy and Law* 14(2):383–403.

Bogue, Richard J., Steven M. Shortell, Min-Woong Sohn, Larry M. Manheim, Gloria J. Bazzoli, and Cheeling Chan. 1995. "Hospital Reorganization after Merger." *Medical Care* 33(7):676–86.

Breyer, Friedrich. 1987. "The Specification of a Hospital Cost Function: A Comment on the Recent Literature." *Journal of Health Economics* 6(2):147–57.

Burda, David. 1996. "FTC Goes to Court to Halt Michigan Merger." *Modern Healthcare* 26(17):22.

Connor, Robert A., Roger D. Feldman, and Bryan E. Dowd. 1997. "The Effects of Market Concentration and Horizontal Mergers on Hospital Costs and Prices." *International Journal of Economics of Business,* in press.

Dranove, David S., Mark Shanley, and Carol Simon. 1992. "Is Hospital Competition Wasteful?" *RAND Journal of Economics* 23(2):247–62.

Dranove, David S., Mark Shanley, and William D. White. 1993. "Price and Concentration in Hospital Markets: The Switch from Patient-Driven to Payer-Driven Competition." *Journal of Law and Economics* 36(1):179–204.

Eckbo, Espen B. 1983. "Horizontal Mergers, Collusion, and Stockholder Wealth." *Journal of Financial Economics* 11:241–73.

———. 1989. "The Role of Stock Market Studies in Formulating Antitrust Policy toward Horizontal Mergers: Comment." *Quarterly Journal of Business and Economics* 28(4):22–42.

Farley, Dean E. 1985. *Competition among Hospitals: Market Structure and Its Relation to Utilization, Costs, and Financial Position.* Hospital Studies Program, National Center for Health Services Research and Health Care Technology Assessment, Research Note 7, Pub No. 85–3353. U. S. Department of Health and Human Services. Washington, D.C., August.

Greene, Jay. 1990. "Do Mergers Work?" *Modern Healthcare* 20(11):24–34.

———. 1992. "The Costs of Hospital Mergers." *Modern Healthcare* 22(5):36–42.

Hay, George A., and Gregory J. Werden. 1993. "Horizontal Mergers: Law, Policy, and Economics." *American Economic Review* 83(2):173–77.

Hospital Research and Educational Trust (HRET), American Hospital Association (AHA). 1993. *Effects of Horizontal Consolidation on Hospital Markets: Executive Summary (R01 HS06250–02)*, Hospital Research and Educational Trust, American Hospital Association, Chicago.

Hughes, R. G., Sandra S. Hunt, and Harold S. Luft. 1987. "Effects of Surgeon Volume and Hospital Volume on Quality of Care in Hospitals." *Medical Care* 25(6): 489–503.

Hughes, R. G., and Harold S. Luft. 1991. "Service Patterns in Local Hospital Markets: Complementarity or Medical Arms Race?" *Health Services Management Research* 4(2):131–39.

Kazemek, Edward A. 1991. "Beating the Odds against Merger Failures." *Modern Healthcare* 21(30):74.

Kmenta, Jan. 1986. *Elements of Econometrics.* 2d ed. New York: Macmillan Publishing Company.

Kralewski, John E., Terence D. Wingert, Roger D. Feldman, Gary J. Rahn, and Thomas H. Klassen. 1992. "Factors Related to the Provision of Hospital Discounts for HMO Inpatients." *Health Services Research* 27(2):133–53.

Luft, Harold S., James C. Robinson, Deborah W. Garnick, Susan C. Maerki, and Stephan J. McPhee. 1986. "The Role of Specialized Clinical Services in Competition among Hospitals." *Inquiry* 23(1):83–94.

Lynk, William J. 1995a. "Nonprofit Hospital Mergers and the Exercise of Market Power." *Journal of Law and Economics* 38:437–61.

———. 1995b. "The Creation of Economic Efficiencies in Hospital Mergers." *Journal of Health Economics* 14:507–30.

Makuc, Diane M., Bengt Haglund, Deborah D. Ingram, and Joel C. Kleinman. 1991. *Vital and Health Statistics: Health Service Areas for the United States, DHHS Publication No. (PHS) 92–1386; National Center for Health Statistics; Series 2, No. 112.* Centers for Disease Control.

Manheim, Larry M., Gloria J. Bazzoli, and Min-Woong Sohn. 1994. "Local Hospital Competition in Large Metropolitan Areas." *Journal of Economics and Management Strategy* 3(1):143–67.

McGuckin, Robert H., Frederick R. Warren-Boulton, and Peter Waldstein. 1992. "The Use of Stock Market Returns in Antitrust Analysis of Mergers." *Review of Industrial Organization* 7:1–11.

Melnick, Glenn A., and Jack Zwanziger. 1988. "Hospital Behavior under Competition and Cost-Containment Policies: The California Experience, 1980 to 1985." *JAMA* 260(18):2669–75.

———. 1989. "Competition Lowers Cost at California Hospitals." *Hospitals* 63(1):56–58.

Melnick, Glenn A., Jack Zwanziger, Anil Bamezai, and Robert Pattison. 1992. "The Effects of Market Structure and Bargaining Position on Hospital Prices." *Journal of Health Economics* 11(3):217–33.

Mullner, Ross M., and Ronald M. Anderson. 1987. "A Descriptive and Financial Ratio Analysis of Merged and Consolidated Hospitals: United States, 1980–1985." *Advances in Health Economics & Health Services Research* 7:41–58.

Noether, Monica. 1988. "Competition among Hospitals." *Journal of Health Economics* 7(3): 259–84.

Perry, Martin K, and Robert H. Porter. 1985. "Oligopoly and the Incentive for Horizontal Merger." *American Economic Review* 75(1):219–27.

Rill, James F. 1992. "An Antitrust Screen for Merger Masters of the 1990s." *Mergers & Acquisitions* 27(2):52–7.

Robinson, James C., and Harold S. Luft. 1985. "The Impact of Hospital Market Structure on Patient Volume, Average Length of Stay, and the Cost of Care." *Journal of Health Economics* 4(4): 333–56.

———. 1987. "Competition and the Cost of Hospital Care, 1972 to 1982." *JAMA* 257(23):3241–45.

———. 1988. "Competition, Regulation, and Hospital Costs, 1982 to 1986." *JAMA* 260(18):2676–81.

Robinson, James C., and Ciaran S. Phibbs. 1989. "An Evaluation of Medicaid Selective Contracting in California." *Journal of Health Economics* 8(4):437–55.

Schumann, Laurence. 1993. "Patterns of Abnormal Returns and the Competitive Effects of Horizontal Mergers." *Review of Industrial Organization* 1993(8):679–96.

Staten, Michael, John Umbeck, William Dunkelberg, and Mark V. Pauly. 1988. "Market Share/Market Power Revisited: A New Test for an Old Theory; Reply." *Journal of Health Economics* 7(1):73–87.

Stenbacka, Rune. 1992. "Mergers, Investments in Cost Reduction and Welfare." *Scandinavian Journal of Economics* 94(1):113–22.

U.S. Department of Health and Human Services, Health Care Financing Administration. 1994. *HCFA Hospital Wage Index Survey* (data sets), Washington, D.C.: USDHHS/HCFA.

U.S. Department of Health and Human Services, Health Care Financing Administration, Bureau of Data Management and Strategy. 1994. *Health Care Provider Cost Report Information System, HCFA-2552-85, PPS II-VIII* (data sets), Washington, D.C.: USDHHS/HCFA.

U.S. Department of Health and Human Services, Office of Data Analysis and Management, Bureau of Health Professions. 1994. *Area Resource File (ARF)* (data set). Washington, D.C.: USDHHS/ODAM/BHP/IARF, September.

U.S. Department of Health and Human Services, Office of Inspector General. 1992. *OIG Final Report on "Effects of Hospital Mergers on Costs, Revenues, and Patient Volume."* Washington, D.C.: USDHHS/OIG, OEI-12-90-02450, July 2.

Vistnes, Gregory. 1995. "Hospital Mergers and Antitrust Enforcement." *Journal of Health Politics, Policy and Law* 20(1):175–90.

Vita, Michael G., and Laurence Schumann. 1991."The Competitive Effects of Horizontal Mergers in the Hospital Industry: A Closer Look." *Journal of Health Economics* 10(3):359–72.

Werden, Gregory J., and Michael A. Williams. 1989. "The Role of Stock Market Studies in Formulating Antitrust Policy toward Horizontal Mergers." *Quarterly Journal of Business and Economics* 28(4):3–21.

White, H. 1980. "A Heteroskedasticity-Consistent Covariance Matrix and a Direct Test for Heteroskedasticity." *Econometrica* 48:817–38.

Woolley, J. Michael. 1989. "The Competitive Effects of Horizontal Mergers in the Hospital Industry." *Journal of Health Economics* 8(3):271–91.

Zwanziger, Jack, and Glenn A. Melnick. 1988. "The Effects of Hospital Competition and the Medicare PPS Program on Hospital Cost Behavior in California." *Journal of Health Economics* 7(4):301–20.

Zwanziger, Jack, Glenn A. Melnick, and Anil Bamezai. 1994. "Costs and Price Competition in California Hospitals, 1980–1990." *Health Affairs* 13(4):118–26.

Index

A Note on the Book

This book was edited by
the publications staff of the
American Enterprise Institute.
The index was prepared by Julia Petrakis.
The figures were drawn by
Hördur Karlsson.
The text was set in Palatino, a typeface
designed by the twentieth-century Swiss designer
Hermann Zapf. Coghill Composition Company
of Richmond, Virginia, set the type,
and Edwards Brothers, Incorporated,
of Lillington, North Carolina,
printed and bound the book,
using permanent acid-free paper.

The AEI Press is the publisher for the American Enterprise Institute for Public Policy Research, 1150 Seventeenth Street, N.W., Washington, D.C. 20036; *Christopher DeMuth,* publisher; *Dana Lane,* director; *Ann Petty,* editor; *Leigh Tripoli,* editor; *Cheryl Weissmann,* editor; *Alice Anne English,* production manager.